Additional Titles From the American Academy of Pediatrics

ADHD: What Every Parent Needs to Know

Autism Spectrum Disorder: What Every Parent Needs to Know

Building Happier Kids: Stress-busting Tools for Parents

Caring for Your Baby and Young Child: Birth to Age 5*

Caring for Your School-Age Child: Ages 5–12

Congrats—You're Having a Teen! Strengthen Your Family and Raise a Good Person

Family Fit Plan: A 30-Day Wellness Transformation

High Five Discipline: Positive Parenting for Happy, Healthy, Well-Behaved Kids

My Child Is Sick! Expert Advice for Managing Common Illnesses and Injuries

Nurturing Boys to Be Better Men: Gender Equality Starts at Home

Parenting Through Puberty: Mood Swings, Acne, and Growing Pains

Protecting Your Child's Health: Expert Answers to Urgent Environmental Questions

Raising an Organized Child: 5 Steps to Boost Independence, Ease Frustration, and Promote Confidence

The Working Mom Blueprint: Winning at Parenting Without Losing Yourself

You-ology: A Puberty Guide for EVERY Body

*This book is also available in Spanish.

To find additional AAP books for parents, visit **aap.org/shopaap-for-parents,** amazon.com/americanacademyofpediatrics, or your favorite bookseller or library.

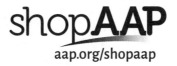

aap.org/shopaap

For more pediatrician-approved advice and the latest updates, visit HealthyChildren.org, the official AAP website for parents.

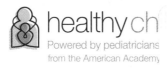

Digging Into Nature

Outdoor Adventures for Happier and Healthier Kids

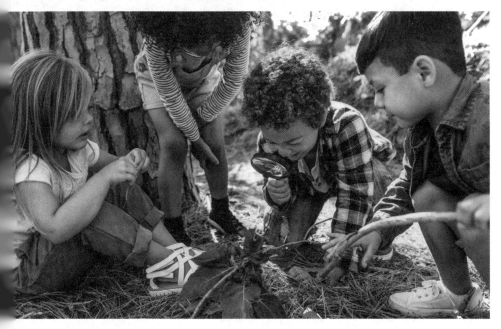

Pooja Sarin Tandon, MD, MPH, FAAP, and
Danette Swanson Glassy, MD, FAAP

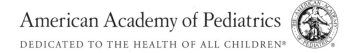

American Academy of Pediatrics

DEDICATED TO THE HEALTH OF ALL CHILDREN®

American Academy of Pediatrics Publishing Staff

Mary Lou White, *Chief Product and Services Officer/SVP, Membership, Marketing, and Publishing*
Mark Grimes, *Vice President, Publishing*
Kathryn Sparks, *Senior Editor, Consumer Publishing*
Grace Klooster, *Editorial Assistant*
Shannan Martin, *Production Manager, Consumer Publications*
Amanda Helmholz, *Medical Copy Editor*
Peg Mulcahy, *Manager, Art Direction and Production*
Soraya Alem, *Digital Production Specialist*
Sara Hoerdeman, *Marketing and Acquisitions Manager, Consumer Products*

Published by the American Academy of Pediatrics
345 Park Blvd
Itasca, IL 60143
Telephone: 630/626-6000
Facsimile: 847/434-8000
www.aap.org

The American Academy of Pediatrics is an organization of 67,000 primary care pediatricians, pediatric medical subspecialists, and pediatric surgical specialists dedicated to the health, safety, and well-being of all infants, children, adolescents, and young adults.

The information contained in this publication should not be used as a substitute for the medical care and advice of your pediatrician. There may be variations in treatment that your pediatrician may recommend based on individual facts and circumstances.

Statements and opinions expressed are those of the authors and not necessarily those of the American Academy of Pediatrics.

Any websites, brand names, products, or manufacturers are mentioned for informational and identification purposes only and do not imply an endorsement by the American Academy of Pediatrics (AAP). The AAP is not responsible for the content of external resources. Information was current at the time of publication.

The publishers have made every effort to trace the copyright holders for borrowed materials. If they have inadvertently overlooked any, they will be pleased to make the necessary arrangements at the first opportunity.

This publication has been developed by the American Academy of Pediatrics (AAP). The contributors are expert authorities in the field of pediatrics. No commercial involvement of any kind has been solicited or accepted in the development of the content of this publication. Disclosures: Dr Pooja Tandon has disclosed a financial relationship as an employee with the Trust for Public Land and an uncompensated relationship as a board member for IslandWood. Disclosures are reviewed and mitigated through a Conflict of Interest process approved by the AAP Board of Directors.

Every effort is made to keep *Digging Into Nature* consistent with the most recent advice and information available from the American Academy of Pediatrics.

Special discounts are available for bulk purchases of this publication. Email Special Sales at nationalaccounts@aap.org for more information.

Shutterstock photo credits: pages 26, 55, 56, and 84. All other photos, unless otherwise stated, used with permission by Danette Swanson Glassy, Benjamin Glassy, Anita Kasina Glassy, Pooja Sarin Tandon, Steven Sparks, Jen Staten, Puneet Tandon, Yogi Sarin, Priya Sarin Gupta, Jaya Sarin Pradhan, Sobia Khan, and Bejamin Aaronson.

Printed in the United States of America

9-509/0924   1 2 3 4 5 6 7 8 9 10
CB0139
ISBN: 978-1-61002-744-1
eBook: 978-1-61002-746-5
EPUB: 978-1-61002-745-8

Cover design by Daniel Rembert
Publication design by Peg Mulcahy

Library of Congress Control Number: 2023948235

What People Are Saying About *Digging Into Nature*

What a good and useful book this is! The tone is perfect for parents, grandparents, and anyone whose life intersects with young children. The information and suggestions are presented in ordinary language, as though the authors were talking directly to you, as though you were a friend. It's actually a perfect gift for prospective parents.

Nancy Pearl, librarian, writer, book reviewer, and author of *George & Lizzie* and the Book Lust series of recommended reading for all ages

Overflowing with useful tips and insightful research, *Digging Into Nature* offers a fun guide for coaxing even the most reluctant children—and their parents—outside and enjoying "green time."

Michaeleen Doucleff, PhD, *New York Times* best-selling author of *Hunt, Gather, Parent*

Digging Into Nature is a book to help parents and children enjoy themselves and each other and the world around them—that is, it's a practical and also inspirational trail guide to finding ways out into nature for *all* children, and thereby enriching their health and well-being.

Perri Klass, MD, FAAP, coauthor of *Quirky Kids: Understanding and Supporting Your Child With Developmental Differences,* and professor of journalism and pediatrics, New York University

Digging Into Nature is remarkable for its source, the American Academy of Pediatrics. It's also remarkable for its attention to the psychological challenges to parents. With kindness and clarity, the authors, both physicians, lead the reader step-by-step through the barriers a parent or another guardian faces when helping children connect to nature. Reading this fine book will serve not only as an informative guide but also as a balm and encouragement to anyone who takes children, and themselves, into the wonderment of nature.

Richard Louv, author of *Last Child in the Woods: Saving Our Children from Nature-Deficit Disorder* and other books about the human relationship with nature

As mothers and pediatricians, Drs Tandon and Glassy share their expertise and passion for getting children outdoors. Through engaging storytelling and practical tips, they inspire parents to prioritize playing in nature for children's mental and emotional well-being. This book is a must-read for parents and pediatricians, especially as a vital alternative to the time children spend on digital media.

> Barry Zuckerman, MD, professor and chair emeritus of the Department of Pediatrics at Chobanian & Avedisian School of Medicine and cofounder of several health initiatives, including Reach Out and Read, Small Moments: Big Impact, Health Leads, and the National Center for Medical-Legal Partnership

A must-read for parents looking for alternative and healthy ways to raise children in a screen-saturated world. It is a beacon of hope.

> Dimitri A. Christakis, MD, MPH, FAAP, chief health officer of Special Olympics International, editor in chief of *JAMA Pediatrics,* and investigator with the Center for Child Health, Behavior and Development at Seattle Children's Research Institute

Needed now more than ever, this book is a prescription for a medicine of the best kind—nature. But far more than a prescription, this book is a guide with tips, facts, and inspiring stories to empower children and families to enjoy time in nature and to understand how easy and important it is to do so!

> Stephen J. Pont, MD, MPH, FAAP, associate professor of pediatrics and population health at the University of Texas Dell Medical School and cochair of the American Academy of Pediatrics Special Interest Group on Nature and Child Health

You would be skeptical, and rightly so, if I told you that I had one effective treatment for a vast variety of common pediatric problems from sleep difficulties to attention issues to maintaining a healthy weight to preventing nearsightedness. What kind of medicine can do all that? I could call it "vitamin N," but honestly, it's just nature.

With *Digging Into Nature,* 2 of my most esteemed colleagues, Drs Tandon and Glassy, team up to guide you and your family on your own personal nature adventure. Along the way, they break down common barriers that limit kids' exposure to nature, from electronic media to bugbites, from water safety to considerations of children with special health care needs. Starting with the cracks in your sidewalk and extending to the blanket of stars overhead, this book will help you serve as your children's best nature guide, no matter where you're starting.

> David L. Hill, MD, FAAP, associate medical editor of *Caring for Your Baby and Young Child: Birth to Age 5*

To all parents, grandparents, and caring adults
who nurture children with an appreciation
for the natural world

Equity, Diversity, and Inclusion Statement

The American Academy of Pediatrics is committed to principles of equity, diversity, and inclusion in its publishing program. Editorial boards, author selections, and author transitions (publication succession plans) are designed to include diverse voices that reflect society as a whole. Editor and author teams are encouraged to actively seek out diverse authors and reviewers at all stages of the editorial process. Publishing staff are committed to promoting equity, diversity, and inclusion in all aspects of publication writing, review, and production.

Contents

Acknowledgments

We are excited for this opportunity to share what we know about nature and children's health with a wider audience. Writing this book was a journey in our learning how to shape information that we typically share with our patients, their families, and our colleagues, for a broader audience.

We owe a tremendous thank-you to our American Academy of Pediatrics editor, Kathryn Sparks. Kathryn helped us present our information in a format and style that makes this book so much more approachable. We appreciate everyone at the American Academy of Pediatrics who was a part of the team that made this book a reality.

We would also like to thank Kelcy Tiger, children's librarian with the King County Library System, for her invaluable help creating the outstanding list of children's books about nature featured in Chapter 7.

We are grateful to our colleagues in the Seattle area and across the country who have encouraged and supported our efforts to elevate the role of nature contact as a way to promote children's health and well-being.

Finally, we both would like to thank the families that have trusted us with the health of their children and taught us so much. We wrote this for you.

Danette Swanson Glassy, MD, FAAP

Guided by all the dedicated teachers and generous mentors, my path to becoming a primary care pediatrician was especially inspired by my very own pediatrician, Dr Joseph Wearn. Thanks to all of these teachers and mentors for nurturing my love of learning and a passion for pediatrics, including all of my practice partners.

In my pediatric practice, I can see how communities, circumstances, and relationships contribute to the well-being of children. I am also grateful to all the child advocates who inspired me to notice and address these complicated issues and to look for answers by stepping out of my office and working for what children and their families need at the local and national levels. My path as a child advocate is nurtured by all the pediatrician volunteers and staff of the Washington Chapter of the American Academy of Pediatrics and the national American Academy of Pediatrics. I thank them all for giving me the most satisfying vocation and avocation. Thanks especially to Dr Edgar Marcuse, who helped me with my first community project as a resident and who has guided our nature and child health work.

I have a very special thank-you for my coauthor, Dr Pooja Sarin Tandon. This book would not exist without her knowledge and creativity. I learned so much, and I am so grateful we have formed this team.

Support from my family has been essential for my professional development as a pediatrician and child advocate. My parents, grandparents, aunts and uncles, and cousins and my brother, David, all made me the nature-loving pediatrician and child advocate I am today. I would especially like to thank my husband, Dr Kyle Yasuda, and my children, Ben, Julia, and Anita. The icing on the cake and my treasure and the most wonderful inspiration are my grandchildren. Thank you to you all.

Pooja Sarin Tandon, MD, MPH, FAAP

During my professional journey from medical school to residency and beyond, I have crossed paths with so many people who have helped me learn that children's health is not determined just by clinics and hospitals but emerges from their families, schools, and communities.

I have been fortunate to be mentored by wonderful physicians, including Drs Sean Palfrey, Barry Zuckerman, Robert Vinci, Dimitri Christakis, Edgar Marcuse, Howard Frumkin, and others, who have nurtured my roles as a researcher, educator, and advocate for child health. I am so grateful to have worked on this book and related work with Dr Danette Swanson Glassy, who always brings so much wisdom and positivity. I am inspired daily by colleagues and trainees at the University of Washington, the Seattle Children's Research Institute, the Trust for Public Land, and numerous community organizations working toward creating healthier, more equitable communities where all children can thrive.

I owe so much to my original nature mentors, my grandparents, and parents, without whose love and guidance I would not be who I am today. I have the best siblings (and nieces and nephews) and friends who have encouraged and joined me in so many joyful experiences outdoors, only some of which I had room to share in these pages. Finally, there's no one I would rather share my life's adventures with than my husband, Puneet, and my children, Akshay and Rishin. I continue to grow and thrive because of your love and confidence.

Introduction

Welcome to *Digging Into Nature: Outdoor Adventures for Happier and Healthier Kids*! We invite all parents, grandparents, caregivers, teachers, mentors, and aunts and uncles and every person who touches the lives of children to feel comfortable in these pages. We want to meet you where you are regarding the role of nature for children's health and inspire you to find more ways to be outside with the children in your life.

As pediatricians, we spend our professional time dedicated to promoting the health of children and know passionately that children thrive with time in nature. Science supports what you may already know intuitively, that time outdoors, especially in nature, is important for the development and well-being of children and can help manage some physical and mental conditions. But in sharing this message with our patients, our colleagues, and our own friends and families, we've learned that even when we know something is good for us, it can be challenging to put it into practice. As parents ourselves, we've been in the position of juggling many roles and priorities, hoping we make the best decisions for our children. In this book, we have tried to compile what we have learned as mothers and as pediatricians with over 50 years of experience between the 2 of us. We provided information on the rapidly expanding evidence-based information regarding nature's preventive care and healing effects. We know many parents for whom the science can be a persuasive force in making changes. The bonus in this book is that we have taken all we have heard about barriers that keep children and their families away from nature and shared practical advice on how to overcome them. And we do this through the lens of promoting better relationships and better health, while admiring the outright magic of time in nature in age-appropriate ways. We also acknowledge that each child, each family, has different interests and circumstances that have an impact on how they access and approach time outdoors. This is not just another nature book for families; this is a nature book for families from 2 pediatricians who have listened to many diverse perspectives carefully and offer research-informed, parent and community–tested advice about the essential childhood experience of nature time.

Who We Are

Danette Swanson Glassy, MD, FAAP: Recently retired from primary care practice at Mercer Island Pediatrics after 32 years, I now spend my professional time on child advocacy. Over the years, I have worked with the Washington Chapter of the American Academy of Pediatrics and the national American Academy of Pediatrics on projects that improved access to health care, increased quality in early care and education, helped schools create anti-bullying policies, and promoted nature and child health. I have a deep appreciation for the Pacific Northwest not only because of the local natural elements but also because my parents and extended family gave me the confidence to explore nature. Our family spent a lot of time in nature, and they also made sure I had time to explore natural spaces on my own. My earliest memories of nature are planned family activities such as camping, fishing, gardening, and collecting, as well as my imaginative play outside. As a young child, I can remember my mom shooing me outside (we were fortunate to have a yard and safe neighborhood) as she told me to "explore." I knew every inch of my 2- to 3-block neighborhood and regularly visited my favorite rocks, trees, and bushes to climb through. My dad arranged big outings, and my mom taught me the names of the flowers and trees that made these natural elements more appealing to me. As my own children grew up, I wanted them to have nature memories too. My most precious nature time as an adult has been watching my own children and grandchildren experience awe during their nature explorations.

It was during a recent patient visit that I became inspired to understand more about nature and time outside on the health and well-being of children. A patient came in for her 6-year well-child checkup. I always ask younger kids what they enjoy outside. This confident kindergartner rolled her eyes and said, "Oh Dr Glassy, I'm not an outdoor girl!" We all laughed, including her parents. We discussed being outside briefly, but it was clear to me that her family prioritized indoor learning, and even computer time, over being outside. These are important things for children to be exposed to but not at the exclusion of nature time. And if a 6-year-old already identifies as "not an outdoor girl," then it's the perfect time to empower families to embrace nature as an important learning environment.

Later that month, a 10-year-old Korean American patient and his mother came with concerns about him gaining weight faster than he was growing. His mother struggled with getting him outside as much as she wanted. As a single mom, she also had trouble finding time for them to be outside. They committed to taking a walk together after dinner once or twice per week. When I saw them weeks later, they reported that on their third time going out for a walk (yay!), a passing driver yelled out that they should "Go back to China" and then slowly followed them for a ways. This heartbreaking encounter scared both of them, and they told me they would not be taking walks together anymore. It was hard for me to realize that this could happen in my community.

For each of these families, the barrier to experiencing nature was very different and surprised me, and each needed support in a different way. I knew I needed to understand more about all the various challenges that keep children out of nature, while offering realistic advice for my patients and their families. This inspired me to work with other pediatricians and child advocates on nature and child health. As I learned more about families enjoying nature with their children, I knew we had much to share about easier access to nature.

Pooja Sarin Tandon, MD, MPH, FAAP: I have been a general pediatrician for more than 20 years, a child health researcher, associate professor at the University of Washington and Seattle Children's Hospital, and health director at the Trust for Public Land. I have conducted studies, published papers, and engaged in various collaborations and advocacy efforts related to the connection between physical activity, time in nature, and children's health and well-being. My inspiration for this work came from a combination of my experiences with my family and what I learned as a pediatrician.

My own connection to the outdoors emerged when I was growing up in India, but I didn't recognize it until many years later, as I didn't grow up hiking, camping, or doing typical American outdoorsy activities. When I was younger, my family did not have tons of outdoor gear and would not have felt comfortable sleeping in tents or sharing bathrooms with strangers. I do remember spending hours playing outdoors in my neighborhood and sleeping under the stars on my grandparents' rooftop terrace all summer long in India. After moving to the United States, I created many wonderful memories of taking walks, visiting parks, and eating outdoors with my friends and family. While I became more comfortable with adventurous outdoor excursions later

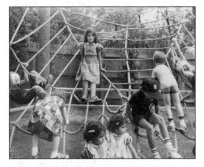

Pooja and her twin sisters when she was young.

in life, I recognize now that my connections with and love for the natural world started early. So, when I became a mother, I think I instinctively gravitated toward prioritizing outdoor time for my children and am grateful we had access to wonderful neighborhood parks, nature-based extracurricular activities, and like-minded friends and family.

As my children got older, I also became increasingly aware of how challenging it was to "make the right decisions" as a parent. I knew I needed to limit screen time but definitely found myself handing them a device to get through a restaurant meal or allow me to work. I debated whether we were overscheduling them with extracurricular activities. Other times, I felt like we weren't doing enough when we heard about some new enrichment class or camp. As the challenges of screen time and hectic schedules became a household reality, I found that we could be healthier, happier, and more resilient as a family when we spent more time outdoors. I intentionally sought out nature experiences for them—as family time, summer camps, and vacations. I even shared life lessons from nature that I know my teenaged children remember today: I had come across a book by W. Thomas Boyce where he discussed "dandelion" children, who were hardy and flourish under most circumstances, and "orchid" children, who were more fragile and needed more special circumstances to thrive. I tried to nurture my children to be dandelions and hoped that including a healthy dose of nature time in their childhood would work toward that goal.

On top of my own parenting endeavors, I was struck by the many, many challenges my patients' families encountered in making healthy choices. Family schedules are busy; healthy options are expensive; and neighborhood conditions vary so much so that driving a few miles can make a huge difference in whether you have safe, accessible outdoor places to play. Parents are balancing so much and trying to do the best they can, and our institutions and systems are not always set up to make healthy decisions easy or equitable. I am grateful to have found a broad community of pediatricians, researchers, nonprofit organizations, and others who appreciate the importance of nature contact for children's health and are working to create, protect, and promote these vital outdoor spaces.

Project Nature

For many years, we have been working together locally and nationally to elevate and advocate for nature-filled childhoods for all children. We have been crafting a successful program for pediatric primary care practices to promote nature time for children: Project Nature (www.projectnaturewa.com). Through this work, we have confirmed that families want nature time for their children, but there can be unique and often overwhelming barriers that keep families indoors and away from the health-promoting natural world. We also confirmed that other pediatricians and pediatric practitioners are eager for tools to support the families in their practices and communities in finding more time in nature. Finally, we have learned from patients, their families, and numerous others about their strategies in creating more nature time for children.

Digging Into This Book

With this book, we want you to find the information about nature and child health that you need so you feel motivated and equipped to provide more nature time for the children in your life.

Our first chapter briefly explores what we mean by *nature time* and the different ways to be in nature. We explain how time in nature can promote health, and we provide an overview of the health benefits for your child in nature.

Chapter 2 is a "deep dig" into the specific health benefits nature provides and connects these to what the current science tells us. You might be surprised by some of our findings, and we hope you share them with others.

We cover some of the barriers our patients have described, or ones we have encountered with our own families, in Chapter 3. For many of the common issues families experience, such as lack of time, weather, lack of access to safe nature, and others, we offer practical suggestions for overcoming these barriers. Our patients have really found this information useful in their own lives.

Chapter 4 is about experiencing nature as children (and families) with special health care needs. This important collection of suggestions is often overlooked in other nature books. Even if you think this information may not apply to your children, we encourage you to read it, as there may be other children in your life or family members facing accessibility challenges for whom this would be useful.

One of the most profoundly humbling and joyful parts of being a parent or caregiver to a child is witnessing their development over time. Chapters 5 and 6 explore using nature time and interactions in the natural world to promote all kinds of developmental milestones and the acquisition of life skills. Each is a thorough discussion of the unique qualities of children at each developmental stage and how that affects their time in nature.

We have collected some of the most inspiring and fun nature activities that we believe are worthy of your limited time in nature in Chapter 7. Each nature activity has suggested modifications to fit the ages of your children, your regional climate, or other special circumstances. In Chapter 8, we wrap up by highlighting international efforts to connect children to nature everywhere and leave you with a message of hope.

Throughout the book, we have sprinkled in pauses for you in the form of the following:

- 🙢 **Reflections:** A prompt to think about how the nature information connects to your life.
- 🙢 **Action Items:** Suggestions for steps you can take to incorporate more nature into your routine.
- 🙢 **Nature Nugget:** Interesting facts, statistics, or studies related to nature.
- 🙢 **Rooted in Culture[a]:** Nature inspiration from various cultural traditions from around the world.
- 🙢 **Ask the Pediatrician:** Questions we've been asked by parents and caregivers.
- 🙢 **Personal Stories:** Inspiring and illustrative stories from our patients, our own families, and friends. We loved bringing the information to life for you in this way.

Our Children and Future Generations

Our hope is that each of you finds something in this book that inspires and supports you in incorporating more time in nature for you and your family. We recognize that we have likely missed questions you have and circumstances you are facing, so we encourage you to check in with your child's pediatrician for additional guidance. We know there are many wonderful ways that you and others around the world have experienced nature, and we look forward to continuing to learn about those.

We hope you will share ideas in this book and invite your family, friends, and others into nature with you. For many people, this is just the opening they need to confidently enjoy nature in a new way, and some children experience nature only through their friends or schools/organizations. We also hope that you seize opportunities to improve nature access in your community and support efforts that work toward more equitable nature access for all. Support your local parks, participate in community cleanups and ecological restoration, promote green schoolyards, advocate for outdoor experiences for all ages and abilities, and vote for leaders who value the natural world. Our children and future generations are counting on all of us.

ᵃWe are neither cultural anthropologists nor members of most of the communities we describe. We share these nature practices and celebrations to offer ideas to enrich your family's nature culture. We know there are numerous other examples, and we encourage you to look for more cultural traditions that will inspire you and your family to enjoy more nature time in new ways.

Chapter 1

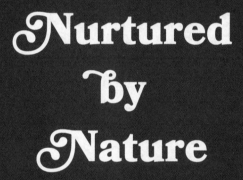

Nurtured by Nature

Nurtured by Nature

Pediatricians think not only about treating illnesses but also about how to support families and communities in raising healthy, happy, and resilient children. During well-child checkup visits, parents often ask us what they can do to optimize their child's health. Just like parents, pediatricians want children to not just have their basic needs met but be thriving. We want children to engage in healthy behaviors that we know are critical for their physical and mental health, now and into the future. There are not many tactics that we as pediatricians can recommend that both promote health and treat diseases. But there is increasing research evidence supporting what many of us already know, that spending time in nature can do both. We believe that contact with nature is an underappreciated, underutilized, and inequitably accessible resource that could ultimately help more children, families, and communities flourish.

REFLECTION: Recall an early childhood memory when you were doing something joyful outdoors. Who were you with? Why was it special?

Depending on where you grew up and what you had access to, you may remember vast natural landscapes or even small pockets of nature that helped you feel calm, curious, joyful, or connected. You may have a memory of an unforgettable nature experience on a family or school trip. Perhaps you had a favorite spot surrounded by nature that you visited often. All children need those opportunities in nature as fundamental childhood experiences. How can we as a community make that happen?

Childhood today looks so different from when you were a child. Like us, you may find yourself reminiscing about how you used to play outside more with friends and family and thinking about how societal trends have affected the way children grow up today. Most children are now spending more time indoors than previous generations, often staring at screens or connecting with friends on a mobile device. Driven by choice or necessity, some children have packed schedules after school and in the summertime, leaving little time for free play in their neighborhoods. Other children don't have access to close, safe places to play or a trusted adult who can accompany them outdoors. In many preschools and schools, opportunities for movement and outdoor play have been diminishing or inequitably distributed. Families, friends, educators, health care practitioners, community members, and others have an opportunity to replenish childhood with nature-based experiences and allow children of all ages to benefit.

All of us can probably think of at least one moment when we experienced a feeling of overwhelming wonder and amazement from something in the natural world. Perhaps it was when you unexpectedly saw the sky painted with a gorgeous sunset or an especially brilliant, low full moon. For me (PT), my first glance into the Grand Canyon took my breath away. As I looked into the vast, rugged canyon that emerged suddenly just steps from the parking lot, I remember feeling overwhelmed by what I saw. For me (DG), the time in nature that sticks in my mind was a beach experience, watching waves repeatedly

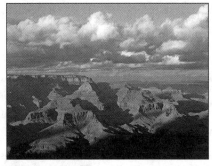

Source: National Parks Service photo by Michael Quinn.

crashing on the rocky shore and listening to the tinkling music as the water retreated back into the Strait of Juan de Fuca. I can still conjure the sight of those powerful waves and the music of the tinkling rocks. We've recognized this look of awe on our own children's faces too, from experiencing immersive, vast nature like a powerful waterfall or a surprise double rainbow to watching a tiny spider spin a perfect web.

That feeling of "wow" that makes us feel like a small part of something enormous is an emotion we are all familiar with: *awe*. There's research suggesting that the experience of awe is related to more happiness, health, and well-being. Are children today receiving enough of those opportunities? The natural world provides a wealth of possibilities for you and your family to experience this sense of wonder, whether close to home or in a renowned natural landscape. We just need to try to prioritize finding those opportunities.

How Does Nature Contact Support Health and Well-Being?

We know there are many ways that nature can boost our health and well-being. When you go into natural settings, ideally you are exposed to fresh air and can move your body, relax your mind, and, if you're there with others, feel joy about spending time with them. Experts have

REFLECTION: Think about a time when you experienced a sense of awe from nature. Where were you, who were you with, and what do remember seeing/feeling?

Nature Nugget: Awe-Inspiring Experiences

Dr Dacher Keltner, professor of psychology at the University of California, Berkeley, writes about how we all need more awe in our lives in his book *Awe: The New Science of Everyday Wonder and How It Can Transform Your Life*. He defines awe as "the feeling of being in the presence of something vast that transcends your current understanding of the world" and suggests we take "micro-adventures" that can provide us with awe-inspiring experiences that are good for our brains and our bodies. He and other scientists have found support for the idea that feelings of awe could bolster our happiness, our sense of connection with others, and even our immune system.

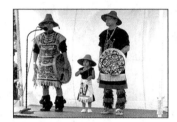

Rooted in Culture

One of my favorite memories is when my husband and I went on a short road trip to a beautiful place called Whidbey Island. We took a ferry ride to get there from Seattle. It was raining the day we planned to go and wasn't the misty rain we normally get but wet, fat raindrops. With rain jackets on, we were delighted to find the Tsimshian Haayuuk dancers from the Tsimshian nations were performing a traditional dance as part of the Penn Cove Water Festival and Native American canoe race. In the pouring rain, we enjoyed watching them. They invited the onlookers to join in. Children enthusiastically began to dance and participate, followed more slowly by others, including us. This will always be a magical experience and memory for us.

—Danette

Tsimshian Haayuuk dancers from the Penn Cove Water Festival.

Source: From the Collection of Island County Historical Society Museum Library and Archives Accession#: 2023.077.002.

proposed different mechanisms for how nature is beneficial for children's health, and we have summarized them into 3 overarching themes.

1. Promotes mental health
2. Supports healthy behaviors and physical well-being
3. Decreases harmful exposures

This chapter explains each of these ideas further, including how they are possible pathways for the connection between nature and health, while Chapter 2 discusses the health benefits of nature contact in more detail.

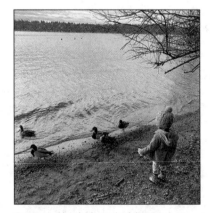

Captivated by ducks at the lake.

Nature Nugget: Defining *Nature* and *Biophilia*

While the most common definition of *nature* refers to plants, animals, the landscape, and other features of the earth and beyond, there is certainly a role for nature-rich spaces created by humans. The term *biophilic design* describes the inclusion of natural elements in the built environment—which includes buildings, schools, parks, and streets—promoting our contact with nature. The word *biophilia* literally comes from the words *bio-*, meaning "life," and *-philia*, meaning "love," and is the basis for a theory that the tendency of humans to feel a connection with and love for nature and other life-forms has, in part, an intrinsic genetic basis.

ACTION ITEM: Think about a built environment setting that you've been to where they've incorporated plants, trees, or other natural elements in a harmonious way. Can you think of a way to bring nature into your home? Maybe you fill a decorative bowl with pine cones or visit a plant store and pick out a houseplant with your child. There are several kinds of plants that are inexpensive and easy for a child to help care for, including succulents, pothos, and snake plants. Some people even name their houseplants and talk with them, which might be fun for your child!

Nature contact promotes mental health

You may have experienced the benefits of going for a walk to step away from a stressful, intense situation to clear your mind. How did you feel before the walk and then after? You may have noticed that taking a toddler outside when they're feeling cranky suddenly changes their mood. For children, recess at school has been shown to have a similar impact in that children return to the classroom better behaved and more able to concentrate on learning. Spending even just a little time near or in nature can increase happiness, decrease stress, restore cognitive capacities, and boost mental health. The capacity of the human brain to focus on something is limited, but it is believed that exposure to nature encourages more effortless brain function, which allows it to replenish its attention capacity.

The scientists who wrote about attention restoration theory explained that natural environments that are immersive and allow us to have feelings of fascination, awe, and escape help restore us. In a study with adults, researchers found that spending even 20 minutes sitting or moving in nature resulted in a 21% decrease in the primary stress hormone, cortisol. Current research doesn't compare the benefits of just being *in* nature with being *active* in nature, but we know that both can help. Of course, if you or your child is also moving in nature, you are also getting a boost from physical activity. Additionally, research suggests that even looking at nature through a window or in photos can create positive emotions and a sense of calm, decreasing stress levels.

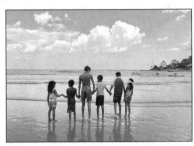
Family reunion at the beach.

ACTION ITEM: The next time you are feeling overwhelmed as a caregiver—there are too many things on your to-do list, or big emotions are making it hard—remember to step outside for just a moment. Notice how the air feels on your skin and in your lungs as you take a deep breath; look for natural beauty, including the sky, and note why that caught your eye. Can you hear some nature, like birds or wind in leaves? What do you smell? If you notice your child becoming overwhelmed, try this strategy with them. As they get older, how wonderful would it be if they learned to use it for themselves when they are feeling stressed?

Nature contact supports healthy behaviors and physical well-being

The movement of our bodies, the blood flow to our brain, and even the company of others while we are moving can be beneficial to people of all ages. Children of any age can experience the freedom to move more vigorously outdoors and in ways that are not always possible, or allowed, indoors. I (PT) remember noticing how excited my kids would be when they got to run, climb, and jump outdoors after spending a long time inside. You've probably seen how young children naturally just start to run or skip when they burst out into a school-yard for recess. While some children seem to become more antsy than others indoors, all children need these opportunities to move freely daily. When children are physically active, they are more likely to sleep

Rooted in Culture

There is a Japanese practice of spending time in a forested space called *shinrin-yoku* or, in translated terms, "forest bathing." Even 20 minutes surrounded by trees is thought to be enough to produce health benefits through the presence of *phytoncides*. These chemicals are natural oils that plants use to defend themselves against insects, bacteria, or fungi and have been found to boost the human immune system by increasing natural killer cell activity. These cells respond rapidly to virus-infected cells and tumor formation. When I (DG) got to speak with Dr Qing Li about his work on forest bathing, he hypothesized that as we breathe in the phytoncides, they cross from our lungs into our blood-stream and then allow our brains to reduce the stress response, lower blood pressure, and act on our immune cells. Studies show that increased natural killer cell activity can last for more than 30 days after a trip to a forest, suggesting that taking a trip once a month would enable individuals to maintain a higher level of natural killer cell activity. The benefits are so well recognized that there are forest-bathing guides, certified in some regions, available to help us reap these benefits from the forest, all over the world. Search online for guides in your area or look for self-guided forest-bathing instructions and head out for a do-it-yourself forest-bathing experience for your family. The Washington Park Arboretum in Seattle has a good self-guided forest-bathing handout and audio guide available on their web-site. The next time you get a chance to venture into a forested space or take a hike among trees, think about all the potential benefits you and your family are experiencing!

better, spend less time on screens, and, over time, have stronger muscles and a healthier weight. Caregivers of the past including aunties and grandmas could have told you that your child will sleep better after hours of vigorous play outdoors, and now we have research to support this idea. Even though physical activity can happen indoors, children are more likely to be active outdoors, especially in nature-rich places like parks. As a pediatrician friend likes to say, "The increased physical activity happens like magic, without extra effort!"

Another way that being in nature helps us be physically healthier may be related to special qualities of the plants themselves. Researchers have found that certain plants (such as pine, cedar, spruce, or fir) give off substances call *phytoncides,* which are thought to reduce blood pressure and boost the immune system, especially if we are surrounded by them in a forest. Being in greenspaces or around animals may increase our exposure to biodiversity, which is increasingly being identified as important for our own microbiomes, or the collection of all microbes, such as bacteria, fungi, and viruses, that naturally live in and on our bodies and contribute to our health and wellness. These microbiomes help our immune system develop, protect us against infections, and assist in digesting food and nutrients.

Nature contact decreases harmful exposures

Most of us have probably experienced harmful environmental exposures such as poor air quality, high heat, and noise at some point in our lives. Air pollution can lead to breathing problems and heart diseases. High temperatures can lead to heat exhaustion and respiratory issues caused by heat-related smog formation. Having forests, neighborhood trees, and other greenspaces can reduce air pollution and create neighborhood environments that are more welcoming and healthier. Take a look around where you live and other places where you and your family spend time. What type of

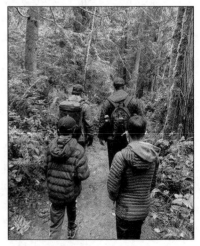

Children and parents on a forest walk.

10

access to greenspaces such as trees and parks do you have near you? If you don't have much, can you think of places you can get to for that type of exposure? Studies from around the world have shown that maintaining and restoring tree cover helps neighborhoods stay cooler, which is critically important in the face of global warming.

Forested areas big and small can provide buffers against noise from traffic and other sources. Children growing up in neighborhoods with less greenspace and parks are exposed to more harmful environmental exposures, compounding their health risks. Living near or spending time in nature or greenspace promotes health by reducing exposure to these harmful elements. Even when we are not aware, our senses register the difference between greenspace-rich environments and environments that lack greenspace. When my (DG) son visited a dense urban setting in the industrial Midwest, he called me with an update. He reported he had traveled just fine but told me "It smells different here." For him, that difference was emotional and triggered homesickness.

Nature Nugget: Trees Are "Cool"

Trees and other vegetation reduce the health consequences of extreme heat. They cool the surface and air temperatures and can decrease energy use for cooling in nearby buildings, by providing shade. Cooling also occurs through transpiration, a process in which trees and vegetation absorb water through their roots and cool surroundings by releasing water vapor into the air through their leaves. In 2023, the US Congress through the US Department of Agriculture has offered $1 billion in grant money to communities all over the country to reduce the human impact of extreme heat by planting trees. This is the most money the government has ever spent on urban and community forests. These grants will prioritize towns disadvantaged by historical injustices and areas of cities that have the least trees and accessible greenspace. This strategy is designed to improve access to nature and improve the health in communities where more than 84% of people live in the United States.

ACTION ITEM: Find out if there is a way for you to support tree-planting initiatives in your community or region or in nearby areas that have fewer trees. Could you and your family volunteer with a community group to plant trees or plant one near your home? There are also national programs such as the US Forest Service Plant-A-Tree program, in which individual donations support reforestation projects across the national forest system.

How Much Nature Do Children Need?

We get this question a lot from parents, and the easy answer is this: children should play outdoors as much as possible! There are more specific recommendations for how much physical activity children should get every day, and these vary by age. For example, the American Academy of Pediatrics and other experts recommend that

- Infants get at least 30 minutes of "tummy time" and other interactive play, spread throughout each day, and outdoor time at least twice per day.
- Toddlers 12 months to 36 months get 60 to 90 minutes of outdoor play each day.
- Kids aged 3 through 5 years get at least 3 hours of physical activity per day, or about 15 minutes every hour they are awake.
- Kids and teens aged 6 through 17 years get 60 minutes of moderate to vigorous physical activity daily.

While all this activity does not need to be outdoors, we know that children are more active when they are outdoors; plus, they benefit in other ways when they are active outdoors in nature-filled settings.

Here's something to remember: there is scientific evidence that even 5- to 20-minute experiences in nature, sometimes called "micro-restorative" opportunities, can improve our mood and decrease stress. So, think of all the ways you can fill your child's nature bucket—perhaps lots of micro-restorative opportunities combined with some that are grander.

Carving out time for nature experiences

We know that most families have busy schedules and are constantly on the go. If you're concerned about finding time in your child's schedule,

Nature Nugget: Good Health in 120 Nature Minutes per Week

It's wonderful when research can support what we already believe, that everyone needs and deserves time in nature. A large study of nearly 20,000 adults showed that people who spent at least 120 minutes in nature a week were significantly more likely to report good health and higher psychological well-being than those who didn't visit nature at all during an average week. These findings were true for men and women, across ages and ethnic groups, among those living in both high- and low-income areas, among those who were meeting physical activity recommendations and those who were not, and even among people with long-term illnesses or disabilities. This study provides at least one benchmark that a minimum of 120 minutes in nature per week is beneficial for our health, regardless of our demographics. And for most children, the more the better!

remember that time in nature can be broken into smaller chunks and can take place in a variety of settings. How does your child get to school? Is it possible for you and your child to walk or bike to school or to the bus stop? If you can walk or bike or ride a scooter instead of driving to school, consider taking a route that has nature surrounding you. You may need to build in extra time and dress for the weather, but many families come to really relish this daily time together. Some families find it helpful to coordinate with neighbors so there is a rotating chaperone for younger children to walk with to school. If before school is not feasible, perhaps you could build in time for a short family walk after dinner during warmer months or, if you have a dog, create a routine for walking your dog together.

It's great to spend time outdoors together with your child, but if you feel comfortable allowing

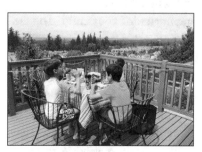
Enjoying snacks with friends on the deck.

them to, older children can experience nature by themselves or with other children. You might encourage your child to take 10-minute breaks on a porch, in a backyard, or in another nearby area, especially if they are getting frustrated with a homework assignment or just need to get through a big project. Another strategy to build in more nature time is to take indoor activities to the outdoors. Think of ways your family may be able to do more things in fresh air, such as reading, homework, art, music, socializing, and eating meals. Perhaps there is a safe outdoor area you can 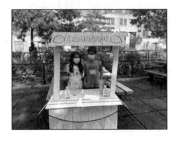 encourage your child to spend time in when they complain that they are bored. Check out Chapter 7 for more age-appropriate ideas and tips on how to get your child outdoors regularly.

Planning for longer outdoor excursions

When schedules allow, longer periods outside are wonderful for more exploration, movement, and connection. For safety and accessibility reasons, younger children rely on adults to take them outdoors, but being in nature together is a wonderful way to spend special time with your older child too. Participating together in a nature-based activity, whether it's a walk or something more adventurous, such as rock climbing, camping, or kayaking, may help parents who struggle to find ways to connect with their tweens or teens. Whether the two of you have deep conversations or both of you savor the quiet time with the family, you are still sharing memorable moments together.

If you have the opportunity to plan family trips to state and national parks or other renowned natural settings, you will create some iconic memories for your child. The US National Park Service has a Junior Ranger program and passport geared toward children aged 5 to 12 years that they can get stamped at all the national parks. I (PT) remember my nieces and nephews being so excited about getting their stamps when we planned a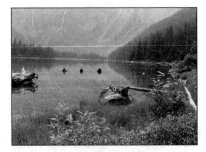

Glacier National Park in Montana.

Happy Nature Birthday!

Having a family whose year is full of winter birthdays, when my younger son was born in July, I was so excited about the possibilities of outdoor birthday celebrations! His first birthday was at a lakefront park with a sandy area, and the children took home inflatable beach balls as their goodie bags. His fifth birthday was at a local farm where kids could pet animals and ride little tractors. We've had celebrations in our neighborhood park, get-togethers in the grandparents' backyard, and a handful of pool parties too. There's a bit of extra logistics involved in trekking party supplies, and there may be more anxiety with closely monitoring the weather forecast, but somehow it has always worked out wonderfully. I've found that you can keep the arrangements simple, that friends and family typically pitch in to help set up and clean, and that the kids seem happier.

Somewhere along the way, we realized it's possible to have outdoor birthdays even in other weather. We brought treats to a covered park gazebo in November and one year did snow tubing with a group of friends followed by hot cocoa. And nature birthdays can be for adults too! I have a wonderful memory of snowshoeing with friends who had me tie a "Happy Birthday" balloon to my backpack, prompting lots of attention and wishes from strangers.

Perhaps you can think about bringing a birthday or another celebration outdoors!

—Pooja

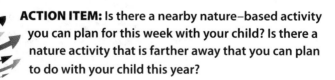

ACTION ITEM: Is there a nearby nature–based activity you can plan for this week with your child? Is there a nature activity that is farther away that you can plan to do with your child this year?

few consecutive family reunions in areas with national parks. The US National Park Service also has the Every Kid Outdoors Annual 4th Grade Pass program where fourth graders (including homeschooled and free-choice learners 10 years of age) receive free access to national parks for that year. One tip we recommend is that if you're hoping to stay within the national parks, it's best to make your reservations early. Many of the national park lodges and campgrounds book up months in advance, and some parks have instituted entry passes that you need to book early. Staying within the park gives you some unique access, like stargazing, watching the sunrise at the Grand Canyon, and the incredible wildlife at sunrise in Lamar Valley at Yellowstone National Park.

It takes a village

Of course, it is unrealistic to expect most parents to be able to take their children outdoors, into nature, every day. We know it can be dark by the time some parents come home, especially during shorter, colder winter days. Many parents have long or atypical working hours, making it even more challenging. We know that evenings can be stressful enough when it comes to making dinner, completing home-work, and getting a bath and bedtime to happen when everyone is exhausted. This is when we suggest you think about all the settings where your child spends time and all the adults who may be able to bring them outdoors. Just as other caregivers help you by ensuring that your child is well-fed, rested, and learning, they can also make sure your child has daily outdoor time. Child care, preschools, and schools can be critical for this since most children spend the majority of their waking hours in one of these places or in the care of someone other than parents.

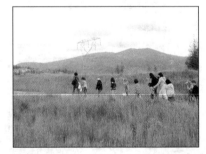

Going on a field trip.

Double-check what your school, preschool, or child care provid-ers' routine is for being outside. Be sure to provide weather-appropriate clothes and sunscreen to help make it easier or more likely that they will take your child outside. Ask for follow-up from their teachers or caregivers about what your child particularly enjoyed and it may inspire new ideas for your own time outside with your child.

Unfortunately, not everyone has easy access to nature-rich spaces that feel safe and welcoming. Picture for a moment a typical school recess occurring on a playground that is all blacktop or concrete with a few plastic play structures. This is the daily reality for millions of children. Yes, these children are still getting a chance to be outdoors, run around, and play with their friends, which are all great for their health and development. Now imagine if their schoolyard is full of nature (some schoolyards are! but unfortunately, not all); they can play with their friends under shady trees, climb on and jump off logs, and check in on their tomato plants in garden beds during recess. In addition to the movement and social opportunities, the natural elements in their schoolyards provide them with cooler temperatures on hot days, challenge their motor skills, and help them learn about ecology. How much nature is in and around the preschool or school where your

Ask the Pediatrician

Q: My school-aged child has recess at school every day. Is that enough nature time during the week?

A: It depends. Some schools have done a great job of "greening up" their outdoor space, so it is more natural and interesting. However, if the recess environment is bare or only on blacktop or concrete, look for other ways to make sure your child has more nature time. If you are interested in bringing a green schoolyard initiative to your local schools or supporting this work for other communities, check out some national movements for green schoolyards that can also serve as community parks after school hours: Green Schoolyards America (www.greenschoolyards.org) and Community Schoolyards (www.tpl.org/our-mission/schoolyards). Either way, be an advocate for daily recess at your child's school and see if there are ways for families and the community to support bringing more nature into those spaces.

child spends time? Does the curriculum include taking children on walks or field trips to natural areas?

Experiencing Nearby Nature

While you can certainly head to the wilderness to immerse yourself in nature, it is comforting to know there are many other ways to connect with and experience benefits from the natural world without traveling too far. We want to emphasize this idea of seeking what we call "nearby nature," which can look very different depending on where you live. But it's these daily possibilities of experiencing the natural world close to where your children live, learn, and play that are so critical and can add up. You and your child could walk a tree-lined street, linger in your child's schoolyard, or spend time looking up at a starry sky. You can closely examine bugs together in the dirt near your home or school. Children have different preferences: some may have a favorite spot under a tree where they like to sit quietly, while others may enjoy playing rambunctiously in a nearby lake with friends and

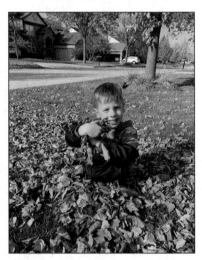

Children can help with yard work and have fun in the leaves!

family. You can take advantage of yard work by having your child help rake leaves and help them notice the changing colors of leaves. You can go on a picnic at the park and discuss fun cloud shapes in the sky. Families do not have to go far or make elaborate plans to spend time in nature. Nature can be found in backyards and neighborhood parks, in community gardens and farms, in schoolyards, and in other public spaces. What other places nearby can you spend time in with your family?

Even observing nature from indoors can be done with little to no preparation. Try observing seasonal changes in trees or phases of the moon from a window, noticing the effects of wind or rain; growing an indoor plant; or organizing a collection of rocks or leaves.

Intentional nature versus incidental nature

Contact with nature can be intentional or incidental, and both have their advantages. *Intentional nature experiences* are those that adult caregivers have more control over. This type of contact could include purposefully choosing outdoor recreational activities for your family such as boating or sledding. How is your child spending time after school, on weekends, and during school vacations?

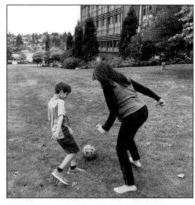

Playing soccer on a college campus.

Are there opportunities for your child to participate in extracurriculars or educational experiences, such as Boy Scouts/Girl Scouts or a gardening club, that would bring them into contact with nature?

Incidental nature experiences happen when your child may be in a nature-rich environment (such as a neighborhood with many parks or a schoolyard with many plants) but is not intentionally there to interact with nature. Consider adding houseplants or moving a desk so your child can look outdoors while studying, for example. Or choose a route through a park or tree-lined street where there's an option to walk places or run errands with your child.

ACTION ITEM: What steps can you take as a parent to increase both intentional and incidental nature exposure for your children?

Intentionally Connecting With Nature

We know you are juggling a lot as a parent, so try your best to build a little more nature time into your child's childhood. With all the possible ways that your child can soak in the health-promoting benefits of time in nature, we are confident that every family can find some that works for them.

Reaping the Benefits of Nature Contact

Reaping the Benefits of Nature Contact

$\mathcal{A}$s parents ourselves, we are always in the position of wanting what's best for our children, but it can be difficult to decide the right thing with so much competition for time and a plethora of recommendations by various experts. In recent years, there has been a tremendous interest in understanding the health benefits of and advocating for nature contact in childhood. The science behind our recommendations in this book is strong, with hundreds of supportive studies. You may be surprised to know that nature contact can not only boost a person's health and well-being but also be part of the treatment of certain conditions. Research shows that there are a wide range of physical,

Nature Nugget: A New Nature Movement

Richard Louv coined the term *nature-deficit disorder* with the publication of his book *Last Child in the Woods: Saving Our Children from Nature-Deficit Disorder,* which describes the increasing human disconnection from the natural world, including its consequences. Louv and others have examined scientific evidence suggesting that when children grow up without sufficient nature contact, this affects their behavior, their development, their physical and mental health, and even their attitudes toward protecting the planet. That term has caught on and fueled an international movement to connect children, families, and communities to the natural world. Louv called for a New Nature Movement, one that recognized the interconnection of all life on Earth, including plants, humans, and other animals. From this call to action, the Children & Nature Network was born and is a wonderful resource for information, strategies, and advocacy on the topic of nature and children. Check out the website (www.childrenandnature.org) for more information.

mental, and developmental health benefits, from prenatal to early childhood years and through adolescence into adulthood. With this knowledge, we hope you will feel that when you make time and space to provide or encourage nature time for your child, your efforts are backed by scientific evidence and guidance from child health experts.

I think back to a very busy time in my (PT) life as the mom of very active 2- and 5-year-old boys. There were not enough hours in the day to get every-thing done, and sometimes those hours were highlighted with exhaustion and self-doubt about whether we were prioritizing the right things as parents. The boys had a lot of energy, and without much intentionality at first, we found ourselves choosing activities outdoors, often with friends. I remember lots of playdates at parks, a Mother's Day picnic at a nearby lake, and short kid-friendly hikes on the weekend. Many things were easier outdoors. I didn't have to worry about one of them knocking over someone's crystal vase, or creating a scene at a restaurant, or getting into a fight over a toy fire truck at an in-home playdate. With less things to break, more space to roam, and new things to explore, somehow there was less tension. Granted, there were the occasional scraped knees, the sometimes unsuccessful last-minute scrambles to find a bathroom, and rocks thrown in the wrong direction. But overall, we felt that parenting was just a little less challenging outdoors.

We were also lucky to be surrounded by people who enjoyed the outdoors and were able to inspire and plan family outdoor excursions that kept both kids and adults happy and entertained. It was on one of these weekend trips with friends to British Columbia, Canada, that I had a revelation of sorts. I had brought a book to read, *Last Child in the Woods: Saving Our Children from Nature-Deficit Disorder,* Richard Louv's work on how the "child in nature is an endangered species" and why this is linked to many of the health problems seen in childhood. It was rare for me to get through more than a book or two per year during those days, but while sitting near the beach on a beautiful day, I looked up and noticed that our children had been digging in the sand, dumping 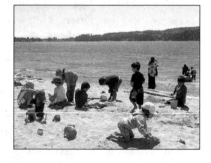 water, building castles, and laughing for almost an hour. No one had cried, no one was hurt, and no one was sad. I read 3 chapters peacefully, rested my body, and nourished my soul. I was sold on this concept of nature-deficit

REFLECTION: Do you already have friends or family that help you and your children enjoy nature? Who could you reach out to for help? Have you been a nature mentor to friends and family, helping them or their children be outside? For more on this topic, see Nature Nugget: Nature Mentors and Allies in Chapter 3.

disorder and decided that as a pediatrician and a mom, I needed to learn more about this topic and do what I could to ensure more nature contact.

Parents, educators, health experts, funders, and leaders often like to see scientific evidence even when some concepts seem obvious or expected. Review studies are a way to compile and critically review evidence from several studies. My (PT) team went through thousands of studies that have been published on the relationship between nature contact and children's health, aggregated what we learned, and published our findings. There are so many different types of studies from around the world focusing on a wide variety of health outcomes that could be influenced by nature contact. Although there are still unanswered questions, there is plenty of evidence to suggest that when children spend time in or near nature, there are many potential benefits and very few downsides.

This chapter features evidence for the connection between healthier, happier kids and nature. Our nerdy families love to understand the connection and strength of the research that goes into parenting advice. My (DG) daughter-in-law said the research references are her favorite parts of this book. Even if you or your family members are not as interested in the science behind our recommendations as we are, you might be surprised by some of the facts in this chapter—and who knows, maybe you'll end up sharing these with others you love!

Prenatal Health

It's common for parents to start to think about their future child's health as soon as they know one is on the way. Expecting parents ask us questions about what to eat and drink, what activities are safe, and how they can support their child's developing brain. Studies have shown that nature contact is beneficial for both the pregnant parent and the baby beginning in pregnancy. Being in or near greenspaces has been shown to decrease symptoms of depression and decrease stress and is associated with better pregnancy outcomes, including higher birth weights and less risk for preterm birth. We were excited to learn that a recent study from the journal *Environmental International* of almost 70,000 births from 11 countries across Europe showed that living near greenspaces was associated with having

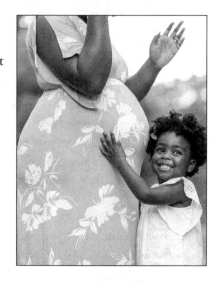

a higher birth weight baby as well as lower risk of birthing a baby considered small for gestational age. Of all the things expecting parents have to think about, it is refreshing to know that science supports taking walks in nature

Complimentary Nature Treatment

I developed high blood pressure during my first pregnancy. At the time, there was not much specific treatment except very careful monitoring, followed by bed rest if it got worse and early delivery if it continued, which is hard on the baby. When I finally went on bed rest, my ob-gyn said the only time I could be up was to use the bathroom or sit quietly outside. Any expecting mother on bed rest knows how (surprisingly) hard it is to just lounge around, day after day. At least a couple of times per day, I would sit in our backyard, all bundled up because it was still cold out, and just watch the trees and birds. This was a nice break from watching too much TV and reading for hours. This quality nature time got me through the long bed rest, and it's reassuring to know that it also probably helped lower my pregnancy-induced high blood pressure. Not only did this nature exposure keep me from getting too antsy, but it likely helped hold off an earlier delivery of my baby.

—Danette

as a way to promote your health and your baby's health. We have personally relished time in nature during our own pregnancies.

During my (PT) first pregnancy, we lived in downtown Chicago and were within walking distance of several parks as well as the lakefront. In addition to packing myself vegetables and nuts for snacks at work and signing up for a prenatal yoga class, I tried to take advantage of my surroundings by going for walks along Lake Michigan whenever possible. During my second pregnancy, heading to the park with my 3-year-old was a great way to keep him entertained too. Taking walks is a wonderful way to move your body during pregnancy, and if you can find opportunities to do so in parks or other nature-rich environments, even better!

Postnatal Health

Of course, once your baby arrives, walking with them in a front pack or stroller can be a nice activity to add to your routine. Depending on your climate, you will need to prepare yourself, but even brief bouts of fresh air can be a helpful distraction from sleepless nights and endless diaper changes. For many new parents, simply going on walks with others can be rejuvenating. My (PT) neighborhood had a Stroller Strides group, which was a full-on outdoor workout group of moms who brought their little ones in tow. Check online to see if something like this exists near you, or create something along these lines yourself with friends who might be willing to join you on a stroller walk or jog on a regular basis.

Nature: The Parenting Solution for More Physical Activity and Sleep

When possible, move your kids outside! The types of movements children can do outdoors are so important for them to develop the movement skills, fitness, and self-confidence to engage in active lifestyles throughout their lives. They can typically move faster and for longer periods outdoors, getting to that higher-intensity vigorous activity that is critical for their cardiovascular and musculoskeletal health. This type of movement is critical because more than 75% of children and adults in the United States do not engage in the recommended amount of daily physical

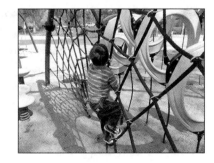

activity. When children learn fundamental movement skills at a young age, such as throwing, kicking, and jumping, they can build on them to do more coordinated movements needed for sports and other active recreation as they grow older. As they practice these skills, they become better at them, and hopefully, they enjoy these activities. It is much harder to pick up a new sport or physical activity as an adult and even as a teenager. But these fundamental movement skills can become the basis for many different types of physical activities, so those people we consider athletic are probably ones who had many opportunities to develop those skills as a child and can more easily pick up new activities.

I (PT) know many adults, especially women, who didn't learn to swim or ride a bike as a child. Some didn't have many opportunities for outdoor, active play because of where they grew up or they didn't learn because of cultural norms for girls in their family. Some of them have now made it a mission not only to model for their children that they can

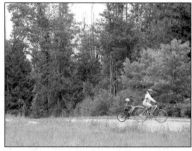

Tandem bike ride.

learn these skills as an adult but also to make sure their children are offered these opportunities early on. We encourage you to do the same, because the childhood years are foundational for helping them develop physical literacy, which is, according to the Society of Health and Physical Educators, "the ability, confidence, and desire to be physically active for life."

Another important concept we want to emphasize and encourage is that there are additional benefits when a child and parent co-participate in a physical activity. Both of you not only gain the benefits of movement but have a

Nature Nugget: Supporting Reluctant Bicyclists

We have had many patients who did not easily learn to ride a bike. Sometimes this was because parents themselves did not know how to ride one either. A great resource found to be beneficial was Pedalheads (www.pedalheads.com). This is an organization available across the United States and Canada that uses a very supportive approach to teach people how to ride a bike safely.

special opportunity to strengthen your bond and build memories. This may be especially important as your child grows and is eager to spend more time with peers. It's an exciting and excellent way to stay connected!

During the COVID-19 pandemic, you may have been one of those parents who took advantage of or even found respite in more opportunities to spend time outdoors with your child. You may live in a neighborhood where you noticed more families taking walks or spending time in the park together. My (PT) research team conducted a national survey study of 1,000 US parents during the pandemic in 2020 and found that more physical activity and less screen time were associated with better mental health for children. We also

Nature Nugget: Walking for Health

Walking is an easy way for most people to participate in physical activity, and you can do it with people of any age. Even many people with disabilities are able to walk or move with assistive devices, such as wheelchairs or walkers. Walking poses a low risk for injury, doesn't require special equipment, has no cost, and is a great way for someone who has not been exercising much to slowly start moving. You can walk instead of taking transportation, for recreation, and even for socialization.

I (PT) come from a family that loves to walk. When I was younger, my grandparents in India rarely skipped their evening walks. Even today, my parents walk almost every single day regardless of the weather. My dad even has an orange reflective crossing guard–style vest that he received as a gift from my aunt and uncle because he is famous for walking even on dark, cold evenings! My sisters and I will frequently go on walks together when we meet up. And I passed this passion of mine along to my children during the pandemic, when we started going on family walks regularly.

If you can't think of another shared outdoor activity that both you and your child would enjoy, try walking! Walk to a coffee shop, walk your dog, or walk on a trail. Walk with friends, walk with colleagues, walk with others from different generations, or walk while talking on the phone with a friend or family member.

Fun fact: Walking at a brisk pace for at least 22 minutes a day allows you to meet the weekly recommendation for adults to participate in 150 minutes per week of physical activity.

found that families that lived within a 10-minute walk of a park reported better mental health among children and parents and more parent-child co-participation in outdoor activity.

Green exercise

Studies support what you probably guessed, that physical activity in natural environments instead of indoors is associated with health benefits that go above and beyond the movement itself, particularly for mental health. Exercising in nature, compared to indoors, has been associated with a better

---

The Importance of Park Activation

I had a 14-year-old patient who loved going to a nearby park to play basketball, but he didn't always feel comfortable being outdoors alone in his neighborhood and his family usually got home too late to go with him. There had been some recent violent incidents near his home. On his own, he figured out the times when other community adults were playing pickleball (a fast-growing racquet sport) in his neighborhood park and he would walk over there to play basketball in the nearby court, during the pickleball practice times, to feel safer. I was so impressed by his problem-solving and was reminded of this idea of park activation.

Just having a public space with sport courts, grass, and trees is not enough to bring people there and, importantly, to help them feel comfortable being there. *Park activation* refers to programming, amenities, and events that allow residents to come together and feel safe and welcome. This can include walking groups, movies or concerts in a park, sports leagues, and the hosting of community and cultural events. Park activation may also support multigenerational park use, which I think benefits everyone from littles to seniors.

This idea also corroborates a study published in 2019 in the *International Journal of Environmental Research and Public Health* concluding that the presence of quality parks and other greenspace reduces urban crime and improves community cohesion. Opportunities for positive social interactions and recreation in inviting, nature-rich public spaces are promising strategies for supporting safer, empowered, more cohesive communities.

—Pooja

ACTION ITEM: Keep a log of physical activity and "green time" for each family member for a week. Older children can help log their hours and will be more accurate about their school and after-school outdoor activities. Are there days when you can add an extra 15, 30, or even 60 minutes of movement outdoors? As a bonus, log hours of sleep as well. Do you notice any differences in sleep quantity or quality (ie, how long it takes to fall asleep or whether it is restful sleep) when there is more physical activity or outdoor time built into your daily routine?

Physical Activity Recommendations

Recommendations for Children Aged 1 to 3 Years
- Be physically active for 60 minutes up to several hours per day in unstructured physical activity.
- At least 30 minutes should be structured physical activity.

Recommendations for Children Aged 3 Through 5 Years
- Be physically active 3+ hours per day for growth and development.
- Adult caregivers should encourage children to be active when they play.

Recommendations for Children and Adolescents Aged 6 Through 17 Years
- 60 minutes or more of moderate- to vigorous-intensity physical activity each day (including before, during, and after the school day).
- Aerobic activity: Most of the daily 60 minutes should include activities like walking, running, or anything that makes their hearts beat faster. At least 3 days a week should include vigorous-intensity activities.

Recommendations for Adults
- Each week, adults need 150 minutes of moderate-intensity physical activity and 2 days of muscle-strengthening activity.
- Some activities are better than none, and it's OK to start with 5–10 minutes a day, a few days a week, and slowly increase.
- We know 150 minutes of physical activity each week sounds like a lot, but you don't have to do it all at once. It could be 30 minutes a day, 5 days a week. You can spread your activity out during the week and break it up into even smaller chunks of time. Try to change your routines to build in more movement: park your car farther away, take the stairs, have a dance party or do stretches with your kids, or meet a friend for a walk instead of a coffee.
- Move more, sit less. Set a timer to stand up and stretch every 30 minutes if you are seated for long periods.

Source: Centers for Disease Control and Prevention. Accessed May 13, 2024. https://www.cdc.gov.

mood, more social interactions, and greater self-esteem, all of which make it more likely that a person will want to do it again. This concept is sometimes referred to as *green exercise,* and even though any physical activity is good for us, why not get that extra boost, if you can, by doing it outdoors?

Nature and sleep

Sleep is necessary for good health, so, as parents, we need to support our children in prioritizing restful sleep. Sleep-deprived children become sick more frequently, are more irritable, and have increased difficulty paying attention in school. Many mental health issues are associated with poor sleep. Parents must ensure that there is an opportunity for younger children to nap, an opportunity for all children and teens to have (screen-free!) wind-down time, and a bedtime that allows for adequate hours of sleep. Ideally, bedtime should be around the same time each night. Figure 2.1 provides the recommended number of hours that kids of various ages should receive. As always, we know that family schedules can get hectic, so do your best to keep consistent family guidelines.

Figure 2.1. Sleep Recommendations
The American Academy of Sleep Medicine provides guidelines regarding how much sleep children need at different ages. Keep in mind that these numbers reflect total sleep hours in a 24-hour period and include nap time. Adults need at least 7 hours per night.

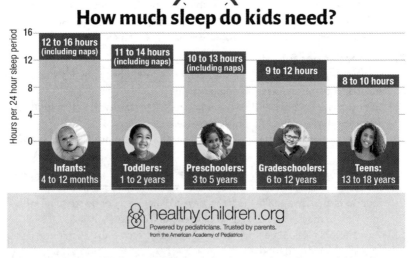

Source: American Academy of Pediatrics. Healthy sleep habits: how many hours does your child need? HealthyChildren.org. Accessed June 14, 2024. https://www.healthychildren.org/English/healthy-living/sleep/Pages/healthy-sleep-habits-how-many-hours-does-your-child-need.aspx and *J Clin Sleep Med.* 2016;12(6): 785–786.

Exploring at Full Speed

My son was 18 months old when it became difficult for him to settle down and sleep during his morning nap. Without good sleep, he was usually crabby and out of sorts, and often his sleep quality was poor during his afternoon nap. One day, while playing outside, he practiced his running in a wide-open space with interesting things to run toward, clearly excited to be able to explore the space at full speed. That afternoon, he took a long, restorative nap. From that point forward, he went outside as much as possible with one nap per day, and thankfully, he had far fewer moments of crabbiness and tantrums!

—Danette

If you have worked hard to create good sleep hygiene for your children, yet they have trouble falling asleep or staying asleep, this can be frustrating. First, try reducing their screen time (especially right before bed, with a screen-free bedroom enforced), and increase their physically active outdoor time during the day. Time in nature can be physically taxing and typically helps children sleep better at night. (See Cell phones + Nature later in this chapter.)

Screen time versus "green time"

Screens are not going away. With our increasing reliance on screens and technology for school and other purposes, aiming for a screen-free childhood may not seem practical. But establishing limits on the quantity and quality of media use outside those requirements, while also encouraging outdoor play, could help mitigate some of the negative consequences. Screen-based media use, including TV, computer, video games, tablets, and cell phones, can have many negative consequences for children's health, including excessive sedentary time, unhealthy weight, and negative impact on development and mental health. We also see children coming into our clinics for neck and back pain as well as sleep issues caused by excessive video game or cell phone use.

According to a review from the journal *PLoS One*, 186 studies examined the psychological impact of screen time and "green time" on children. In this review, *green time* was broadly defined as time spent in, or exposure to, natural environments, elements, or content. The article concluded that screen time was indeed associated with negative psychological impacts and green

Rooted in Culture

Many Nordic countries, including Norway, Sweden, Denmark, Finland, and Iceland, prioritize time spent outside, especially for children and families. There is a long history of improving child health through outdoor exposure and activities. Many Nordic people refer to this priority as *friluftsliv*, meaning "open air life." It is about noncompetitive, nonmotorized outdoor exploration together in nearby nature and finding joy in the process.

This cultural priority extends to the practice of having babies nap outside, year-round. Many parents in these countries believe that the fresh air promotes growth and that the baby sleeps better. Danish child care sites often have areas designated for outdoor naps, and all the Nordic countries have long had outdoor preschools where young children spend their entire school day outside, year-round. If you're worried about taking your little one outdoors, take inspiration from this Nordic tradition and know that if your baby is dressed warmly, they can certainly be outdoors, in most weather.

ACTION ITEM: Introduce the concepts of screen time and "green time" to your family. Can you come up with some family rules together to limit screen time and increase family green time? Families in our practices often struggle with how to start limiting screen time. Universally appreciated was the step-by-step advice given in the American Academy of Pediatrics guide to creating a Family Media Plan. This is practical and detailed advice to making a Family Media Plan (www.healthychildren.org/English/fmp/Pages/MediaPlan.aspx).

time had positive impacts on mental health, cognitive functioning, and academic achievement.

Some suggestions for limiting screen time include

- No screens during meals.
- No screens in bedrooms (especially overnight).
- Screen-free family times prescheduled during the week.
- No screens during car rides of less than 30 minutes.

- No screens during gatherings with friends/playdates.
- Set up limits on phones and tablets so they automatically turn off certain apps after a certain amount of time, or use other technology that limits time.

Some suggestions for family green time include

- Preschedule a family outdoor activity every week and rotate who chooses (the activities will be different depending on climate and season).
- Eat a meal outdoors, if possible.
- Walk a pet together a few times per week.
- Schedule regular 1:1 special time where your child picks the green time activity.

One parent I (PT) knew had a rule that her child had to earn screen time by spending time playing outdoors: 30 minutes outdoors meant 30 minutes of screen time. During the pandemic when my children were doing remote schooling from home, I used a whiteboard to make a daily list of activities they had to complete before screen time, such as schoolwork, chores, and 60 minutes of outdoor time. These types of rules or arrangements may not work for every family, but setting up some guidelines about completing other tasks before screen use is a good strategy. Writing down expectations for your child is a handy parenting tool that helps children and parents be in agreement on what should get done in a day.

Limiting cell phone use

If your child is old enough to have a cell phone, remember to have these discussions about family rules before they receive their phone. You might consider teaming up with your friends and families for additional support. There are national campaigns such as Wait Until 8th wherein parents sign a pledge to delay getting a smartphone for their child until the end of eighth grade to protect middle schoolers from the distractions and dangers of having their own phone.

Some families will choose to buy their child a basic phone that allows only calls and texts, or a smartwatch, if they need a means for communication. We know that for children who spend significant time between 2 homes, this can be very helpful. Another strategy is to have a "family cell phone" that your child can borrow for use when it seems necessary, such as when coordinating pickup after events or during times they'll be away from you for extended periods. This can provide you and your child peace of mind when you need

Nature Nugget: Screenagers

Filmmaker Dr Delaney Ruston is also a physician who has made some incredible documentaries and set up resources for families to understand the impact of screen use and solutions to try to find balance. *Screenagers: Growing Up in the Digital Age* and subsequent films that address youth mental health and substance use in the digital age are powerful and could be beneficial to watch with your older child. Many schools have hosted screenings of these movies, and you could talk with your school leaders about that possibility. You can also check out her weekly blog with practical tips on facing all kinds of screen-related challenges as parents.

Check out the film site too (www.screenagersmovie.com).

to be able to reach them but doesn't give them unrestricted access. There are also phone features and apps you can explore that limit duration of use and the types of content they can access. If your child already has a phone or other electronic devices (eg, computers, video gaming systems, tablets), it's never too late. Talk with them about the dangers of excessive or inappropriate screen use and ask for their ideas on how you can all engage in healthier media use. You may be more successful in changing household patterns and habits if everyone has a chance to provide input and is in it together.

Cell phones + nature

So how does a smartphone relate to nature? Are there phone apps that can be used outdoors that could potentially increase connection with the natural world? The answer is yes! There are apps available that can help you and your child identify plants or bugs just by taking a photo of them. There are also ones for identifying birds through a photo you take or through a birdsong you record, and others show you planets and constellations when aimed at the night sky. There are ones that help you find trails and hikes and include the option for users to input comments about conditions and photos. There are even apps that can help you track your green time. One we found is called 1000 Hours Outside, where they provide tips and inspiration to have your family spend 1,000 hours outside per year (www.1000hoursoutside.com). If you use ChatGPT or a similar generative artificial intelligence platform, you can use it to get ideas for nature activities. Try prompts such as "Create a nature scavenger hunt for a 5-year-old" or "What are nature activities a 9-year-old can do in the rain?" While using screens to promote green time may seem contradictory, we are supportive of minimal but appropriate use of these technological advancements, as we think they can help inform and connect us to nature. You could even use this as an opportunity to talk with your child about appropriate and selective use of certain apps and technologies.

At every well-child visit, we aim to talk with our patients and their families about how all our movements over a 24-hour period connect to each other: physical activity, screen time and other sedentary time, and sleep. For example, a toddler or preschooler who is still taking long afternoon naps may have difficulty falling asleep for the night at a desirable hour. We might suggest limiting their nap time and/or making sure they are awake from their nap by 2:00 or 3:00 pm, and then spend some time playing outdoors in the late afternoon to help with bedtime. An all-too-common example of how these movement behaviors relate to each other is when we hear about so many older children who are not sleeping enough and are tired during the day. We usually emphasize turning off screens (including phones!) for at least an hour before bedtime to receive better quality sleep. Partaking in enough movement and exercise during the day, and limiting screen use (especially before bed), is important for all of us.

Healthy Weight

As pediatricians, we monitor children's growth at every checkup, including their height and weight. While there is a range of healthy weights, we know that having overweight or obesity can put children at risk for additional health problems in childhood and later in life. In our clinics, we focus on the message of healthy lifestyle choices and making those choices as a family. In addition to counseling about healthy nutrition and movement, we encourage children to spend time in parks and greenspaces as a way to promote not just healthy weight but overall well-being. Studies show that children who lack access to parks or greenspace in their neighborhood are more likely to have overweight or high blood pressure. This information about health disparities can be used by community members to advocate for building and maintaining parks and making them welcoming environments for all children and families.

There are examples from around the country where community collaborations have led to the creation of parks, trails, and other greenspaces. One example from Colorado is RISE Southeast, a resident-led organization that partnered with the City of Colorado Springs and the Trust for Public Land to address the lack of safe outdoor spaces in their community. With community input, a 13.5-acre previously unwelcoming space was transformed into a reimagined Panorama Park with an accessible playground, sports courts, splash pad, fitness station, and community spaces with art installations for this neighborhood's 70,000 residents, including 3,350 people who live within a 10-minute walk.

In Chicago, the Bloomingdale Trail (once a train line), known to many locals as The 606, took a decade to be created. One of the neighborhoods in the city, Logan Square, had the least amount of open space per capita in the city, so residents gathered to discuss best ways to change this fact. Dozens of groups, including the Friends of the Bloomingdale Trail, the Trust for Public Land, the Chicago Park District, and many more, were instrumental in the planning, support, and implementation of the project. According to the website (www.the606.org), "The 606 brings together arts, history, design, trails for bikers, runners, and walkers, event spaces, alternative transportation avenues, and green, open space for neighbors, Chicagoans, and the world."

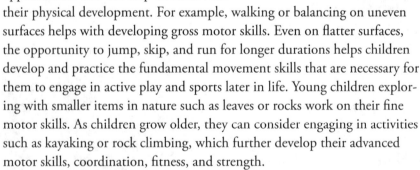

Child Development

Outdoor, nature-based activities offer many opportunities that can help children with their physical development. For example, walking or balancing on uneven surfaces helps with developing gross motor skills. Even on flatter surfaces, the opportunity to jump, skip, and run for longer durations helps children develop and practice the fundamental movement skills that are necessary for them to engage in active play and sports later in life. Young children exploring with smaller items in nature such as leaves or rocks work on their fine motor skills. As children grow older, they can consider engaging in activities such as kayaking or rock climbing, which further develop their advanced motor skills, coordination, fitness, and strength.

Risky play

Hear us out: despite the desire to keep our children safe, we as parents can't prevent our children from experiencing all harm. Playing in nature offers

Observations From an Urban-Located Preschool Teacher

Many years ago, I met a preschool teacher who shared what she had observed about children coming to her urban preschool. Her wisdom has been echoed over the years by other early childhood educators and those who study children's play.

At the beginning of the school year, there is often a lot of interest in the slide play structure. Children climb up the predictable, equidistant steps of the blue ladder, and then they celebrate their ascent to that top briefly, before launching off onto the yellow slide and back to the ground. As the play period progresses, the up-the-ladder-down-the-slide routine starts to feel less fascinating. Children then look to other activities—digging, building, or exploring—in the natural areas to keep their interest. The exciting thing about natural elements, like leaves, rocks, sand, sticks, and acorns, is that there are infinite ways to be creative and play with them!

There is even a theory of loose parts developed by Simon Nicholson in 1971 that explains how materials that can be moved, carried, combined, and taken apart and put back together in multiple ways can empower a creative imagination. The more materials and individuals involved, the more ingenuity that takes place.

This preschool teacher also mentioned she could often tell at the beginning of the year those who had engaged in more outdoor play versus those who had not. Most children were comfortable on the play set, but after a while, there was little challenge and thrill. She could even tell from their unease that some children had never walked on uneven surfaces like the dirt piles the preschool had or climbed up on a log with the knots and roughness. But each time they did, it was potentially different, creating a unique experience and learning opportunity. Climbing the log from the other side or when it's wet can be a whole new challenge for a 3-year-old.

She recounted how one little girl refused to walk on the grass! This teacher learned from the parents that the girl had never walked on grass before and just didn't like how it felt. At first, I was shocked that this little girl had reached the age of 3 without ever having walked on grass. But then I thought about all the reasons that could have led to this, especially living in a large urban area where there may not have been a lot of grass nearby or not have been many opportunities for a busy parent to expose their child to these experiences.

—Pooja

children the opportunity to engage in *risky play*, which is typically defined by child development experts as exciting play experiences or activities that could pose a slight risk to a child's safety. Examples of this include climbing a tree, using some more advanced tools, or engaging in rough-and-tumble play. While this may seem like an uncomfortable idea at times if you haven't tried this yet, remember that giving children the opportunity to engage in challenging experiences allows them to test their own limits and learn. Of course, should you allow your child to engage in this type of play, start any sort of riskier play activity with adult guidance and supervision and then work up to more independence. A related concept adopted by Girl Scout camps is Challenge by Choice, wherein facili-

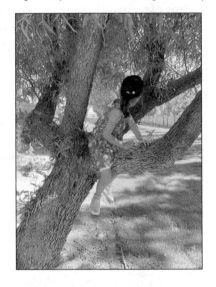

tators offer physical and psychological challenges to participants, but they can choose their level of engagement in the particular challenge.

It took me (PT) a while to become comfortable as a parent letting my boys engage in some riskier play activities, whether that activity be climbing higher on a tree, taking a more challenging route on a hike, or jumping off a taller rock. When they asked for permission, rather than say no right away, I calculated the risks in my mind. With a supportive hand (and always with ground rules), I began letting them test the boundaries. Even when they couldn't reach as high as they had hoped, my children seemed satisfied that they had the chance to try. Afterward, they'd continue to make a few more attempts and often eventually succeeded. Just as I wanted them to remain curious and take intellectual risks as they grew older, it was important for them to take some physical risks and learn the versatility, power, and limits of their bodies.

Risky play can also help children practice regulating their emotions, such as fear or anger, when they are faced with a new challenge. They may need to overcome some hesitation at trying a new activity or frustration when they don't accomplish what they are hoping to on the first try. Through this type of play, they learn how to work through those strong feelings in other situations. By engaging in riskier play, children can learn how to keep themselves safe, potentially resulting in fewer, not more, injuries. If they learn

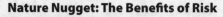
Nature Nugget: The Benefits of Risk

The National Association for the Education of Young Children, a professional membership organization that works to promote high-quality early learning for all young children, birth through age 8 years, encourages early childhood educators to reframe their views of risk-taking by acknowledging the developmental benefits of taking risks and working to remove barriers and boundaries that limit open, free play.

According to the website, "While acknowledging that risk taking is developmentally appropriate and a healthy part of early childhood, educators often find themselves in a paradox: they want to foster risky play and urge children to step out of their comfort zones, but they also must ensure safety. Knowing when to intervene can be challenging."

Their guidance on when educators should insert themselves into risky play situations instead of allowing free play aptly applies to parents as well.

- The level of risk could lead to serious injury.
- A child demonstrates emotional distress or fear.
- The structure or environment is hazardous (eg, ice on play surfaces, broken glass, construction).

to climb up and down a low tree safely, they are less likely to get hurt on subsequent tries. We could also argue that participating in sports is a type of risky play that many parents are comfortable with, despite the risk for injury. Even spending time outside at night or in different weather conditions—hot, cold, windy, or wet—exposes children to variations that help them build up resilience and learn how to be prepared for circumstances that they cannot predict or control.

Child-directed and adult-directed play

When children choose how they play outdoors, they learn to be creative and problem-solve. They may have to negotiate and make compromises with their friends. You might remember coming up with your own games or your own rules while playing at outdoor recess or in a neighborhood or park. I (PT) have fond memories of playing with neighborhood friends of all different ages when I lived in India with my grandparents. I don't remember the details of how we came up with our games or rules, but I knew we had such a variety of activities—from

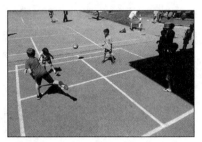

Child-directed play is beneficial to your child's development.

variations of games of chase, to hopscotch, to elaborately planned weddings for our dolls. I especially valued that there were older children who looked out for us, and we figured out how to encourage and include the younger children. We've heard from friends and colleagues about their memories of being allowed to play unsupervised in their neighborhood until dinnertime. We realize that this may not be the reality or even a possibility for many children today, but consider if there are times when you could provide these opportunities for your child. The most reliable opportunity for child-directed play is probably school recess, so make sure to be a fierce advocate to keep that opportunity available to children. Child-directed play is an important developmental opportunity, especially during a time when many children's

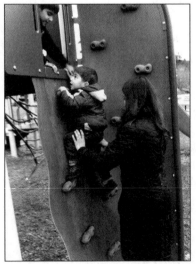

Allow your child to engage in risky play with adult supervision.

activities are adult designed and adult led and often occur with children from the same grade or age-group.

Of course, being outdoors with a trusted adult is also beneficial, so children benefit from both child- and adult-directed play opportunities. Parents or teachers can teach them skills and support them in trying something they haven't experienced before, such as identifying a certain plant or bug or navigating steeper or slippery terrain safely. They can help make sure children are included and supported in ways they need in order to try a new outdoor challenge. And when children experience nature with a parent or another caregiver, they build those important relationships, and that encourages healthy physical and social-emotional development.

Mental and Behavioral Health

As pediatricians, we unfortunately sometimes have to diagnose children with depression or anxiety and certainly see many children who report persistent feelings of sadness and hopelessness. Psychotherapy and medication are sometimes prescribed and often just part of the treatment plan. But we also like to focus on lifestyle factors that can help children manage these difficult emotions and build up their resilience. We want to equip our children with as many strategies as we can to help them deal with life's ups and downs and the inevitable challenges they may face. These lifestyle factors come down to the basics of encouraging getting healthy sleep, eating well, moving their bodies, and spending time with others who bring them joy. Time in nature easily checks off many of those boxes and can be a core part of helping a child or teen on the road to recovery from mental health challenges.

The studies that have shown positive relationships between nature and mental health frequently do not rely on faraway, "big" nature. In fact, nearby parks, trails, gardens, and backyards may be enough of a "dose" to help children gain mental health benefits from nature. Other studies have looked at the impact of immersive wilderness experiences and shown them to be helpful, especially for more significant mental and behavioral health problems,

Nature Nugget: Exploring the Healing Benefits

A study from South Korea investigated the impacts of forest-healing programs on the psychological health of children in foster care. About 4,000 children (middle school–aged or older) who were in foster care in South Korea participated in a program offered by the National Therapy Forests and National Center for Forest Therapy. Most of the children lived in shelters located in urban environments. Self-report surveys completed before and after the program showed a statistically significant overall increase in interpersonal relationship skills, including friendliness, sensitivity, openness, and communication, for these children.

Source: Hong J, Park S, An M. Are forest healing programs useful in promoting children's emotional welfare? the interpersonal relationships of children in foster care. *Urban For Urban Green*. 2021;59:127034.

Nature Nugget: Nature as a Stress Buster

California's former Surgeon General Dr Nadine Burke Harris issued a report in 2020 called *Roadmap for Resilience: The California Surgeon General's Report on Adverse Childhood Experiences, Toxic Stress, and Health.*

Adverse childhood experiences, or ACEs, are potentially traumatic events that occur in childhood and include things such as witnessing or experiencing violence and growing up in a household with substance use problems or food insecurity.

ACEs are linked to chronic health problems, mental illness, and substance use problems in adolescence and adulthood and are common; approximately 64% of US adults reported they had experienced at least one type of ACE before age 18 years. In this report, they (Harris and colleagues) identified 7 healthy ways to manage toxic stress—now referred to as "stress busters"—and fortunately, access to nature is one of them.

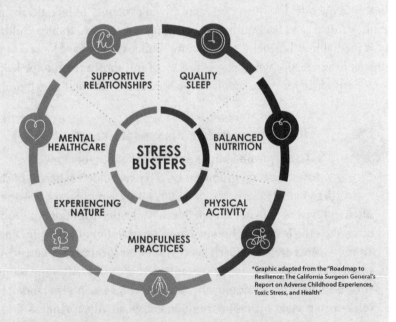

SUPPORTIVE RELATIONSHIPS

QUALITY SLEEP

MENTAL HEALTHCARE

STRESS BUSTERS

BALANCED NUTRITION

EXPERIENCING NATURE

PHYSICAL ACTIVITY

MINDFULNESS PRACTICES

*Graphic adapted from the "Roadmap to Resilience: The California Surgeon General's Report on Adverse Childhood Experiences, Toxic Stress, and Health"

Source: ACES Aware Family Resilience Network, California Department of Health Care Services, Office of the California Surgeon General. (2023). *Stress Busters.* Aces Aware. Retrieved from acesaware.org.

including substance use disorders, technology addiction, school refusal, major depression, and posttraumatic stress disorder. If someone in your life is struggling with one of these conditions, look into these wilderness therapy programs to help. There are also organizations like Wild Grief (www.wildgrief.org), based in Olympia, WA, that provide free peer support for children, families, and teens experiencing grief after the loss of a loved one through hiking, camping, and backpacking trips.

The mental health consequences of climate change are increasingly being recognized, with young people particularly affected. Certainly, there are direct psychological impacts of climate disasters such as wildfires, hurricanes, tornadoes, and floods. But even without direct exposure, young people can be distressed about the ongoing global environmental crises. *Eco-anxiety* or *climate change anxiety*, defined as a state of emotional and mental distress brought on by drastic, negative changes to the environment caused by the warming of the planet, has been identified in children as young as those in elementary school. Helping children connect to efforts to restore the environment, through their

Nature Nugget: Our Planetary Health

When children spend time in nature, it is not only good for their health but good for our planet's health. As we increasingly recognize the impact of human behaviors on the earth, it becomes imperative that we nurture the next generation of environmental stewards. We are much more likely to care about something when we feel connection and value. Research shows that spending time in nature helps children develop pro-environmental attitudes and behaviors and a sense of connection with the natural world. For example, after spending time in nature, children may be more likely to want to recycle or compost materials, conserve electricity and water, or reduce car trips.

Potentially more impactful than recreational outdoor time is when older children engage in ecological restoration, such as helping remove invasive plants or planting trees, to restore degraded or destroyed ecosystems. Ecological restoration not only repairs our natural environments but also has been seen as a public health intervention given what we know about the benefits of nature for human health.

ACTION ITEM: Many schools now include opportunities for children to learn about and engage in environmental education and ecosystem restoration. Ask if your child's school has these opportunities. You can also explore after-school or summer opportunities where children can work with local organizations committed to ecological conservation and restoration. Your child may develop a special connection and feeling of responsibility when they clear a habitat, pick up trash, or help plant trees or a garden. Many community groups, including Native American and other Indigenous groups, sponsor these efforts as well.

Managing ADHD With Less Medication

I was fortunate to care for a patient with attention-deficit/hyperactivity disorder (ADHD) not only in childhood but well into their college years. Her symptoms limited her success in school, but thankfully, ADHD medications were helpful for her learning. In college, with fewer lecture hours, and dedicated time for studying, she began to think about how to manage her attention without medications that were active all day. She scheduled a checkup with me at the end of her first semester to discuss modifying her medication regimen. She was beaming and so proud of what she had discovered. When studying, she set a 15-minute timer, and when it went off, she went outside for a few minutes. She found she was able to manage the necessary focus on even the "most boring" studies if she added in nature breaks. She was successful even with significantly reduced medication.

—Danette

---

school or community programs or even informally as a family, can be good for so many reasons. Children actively engaging in ecological restoration could not only experience benefits to their health but also start to see themselves as part of a solution to negative changes in the world.

There is also compelling evidence that time in nature helps with symptoms of attention-deficit/hyperactivity disorder (ADHD). Studies have shown that after spending time in nature, children with ADHD are able to concentrate better to complete tasks. Anecdotally, teachers report that sometimes their students who have more behavioral challenges with classroom expectations thrive well during outdoor field trips and environmental education opportunities. With the freedom to move and explore in ways that are not possible or encouraged indoors, these students may especially benefit from learning opportunities outside the confines of a building. One family shared with me (PT) that their child's school performance and home behavior improved significantly when they moved to a new home where their child with ADHD spent much more time outdoors. Other families have found success with putting a timer on for 20 or 30 minutes while their child with ADHD is doing homework to schedule short breaks for them to wander to the backyard or porch to regain focus. Even for children who do not have a formal diagnosis of ADHD, helping them learn a strategy of taking a nature break or walk as a way to clear their mind can give them a skill that many adults find useful.

Vision

You might be surprised to learn that there is considerable research and support for the idea that time outdoors is beneficial for children's vision. According to a review in the *Journal of Ophthalmology* from 2016, with about half the world's population expected to be myopic, or nearsighted, by the year 2050, this vision research has significant implications for population health. More than 50% of my (PT) extended family already wear glasses or contact lenses! Experts suggest that time in sunlight, more vitamin D, and a break from focusing on things such as screens help prevent the development and progression of myopia. Studies show that children who spend 40 to 60 minutes outdoors each day can reduce their risk of developing myopia. Of all the reasons to encourage your child to play outdoors, add vision to that list and know that some children may not end up needing glasses or could delay their need for glasses because they spent more time outdoors!

Additional recommendations include taking regular breaks from screens to minimize eyestrain. Have you heard of the 20-20-20 rule? You can teach your child and practice this yourself: every 20 minutes, shift your eyes to look at an object at least 20 feet away, for at least 20 seconds. Ideally, use that 20-minute mark to stand up to take a break from being seated, and look out a window, especially if you have one that provides views of nature.

Remember to protect children's eyes from harmful UV rays when they are outside. Ophthalmologists recommend that even infants wear sunglasses made for their size, but if that proves challenging, you can opt for a hat or other gear that provides a wide brim for shade. We recognize that this is not common practice when children are playing outdoors at recess or during sports, but it's important to know that UV damage to the eyes is cumulative and children's eyes are even more vulnerable than those of adults.

Asthma and Allergies

Since we discuss the range of scientific evidence, it is important to mention that there are some aspects of health that could be negatively affected by certain types of contact with nature. For example, the studies on asthma and allergy symptoms featured mixed results, some showing reduced symptoms with more greenspace or nature contact and others showing more symptoms. That doesn't mean that children with asthma or environmental allergies should not enjoy the outdoors; it just means that they may have to take some extra precautions. We certainly see some patients experience an increase in their allergy and asthma symptoms during times of high pollen count or after they've spent long periods in certain outdoor settings. This may vary depending on the types of allergies they have and how much pollen exposure they get. There are also internet resources, often linked to weather sites, that have local information on daily pollen counts that can help you plan if you know your child's specific allergies. Parents who have children with asthma and environmental allergies can also talk with their child's pediatrician about

Don't Let Allergies Slow You Down!

My younger son has significant allergies to grass pollen... and he's a multisport athlete! This means that springtime soccer can be especially rough on him if we are not extra careful. He knows that when he comes home with red, itchy eyes and a cough after practice, I'm going to ask him whether he's been taking his medications. I remind him to jump into the shower right away and not to lie down on his bed with his pollen-covered clothes. The same kinds of things happen if he's at an outdoorsy summer camp or we spend a long day at a park. These environments haven't stopped him from playing soccer or participating in outdoor events, but they do trigger his allergies. He's old enough now that he makes sure he has his "pharmacy" of allergy tablets, eye drops, and a nose spray that keeps him as healthy as possible.

—Pooja

strategies, including medications and environmental controls, to keep their symptoms under control so they, too, can participate in nature-based and outdoor activities safely.

We've had patients who are able to participate in outdoor activities, sports, or camps without problems if they stay on their prevention medications and shower (for those with pollen and other environmental allergies) right after coming indoors. We know that all children need time in nature, so it's a matter of preparing and tailoring their experience, so they stay healthy and comfortable during and after spending time outdoors.

Nature Improving Parents' Health

While we are focusing on children's health, it is important to point out that nature contact is beneficial to the physical, mental, and cognitive health of adults as well. The research on benefits for adults covers an extraordinary list of conditions, including obesity, cardiovascular disease, diabetes, depression, anxiety, and stress. Parents recognize deep down but sometimes forget that being healthy ourselves can help us parent better. When you feel physically and mentally well, you can participate in more activities and be better engaged with your child, including modeling healthy habits. We have heard that for some parents, especially those who have children with behavioral or learning challenges, spending time in nature together helps both of them feel calmer and enjoy each other's company in ways that can be difficult indoors or in settings with more restrictions. For parents of tweens and teens, it can be refreshing to find a new outdoor activity to do together or continue a childhood tradition as a way to stay connected with your child during a developmental stage when they strive to be more independent.

Taking care of your mental health as a parent is essential, as it has such an impact on your child and family. We both know parents who have turned toward nature activities as self-therapy during particularly challenging times in their lives, including going through a divorce, caring for a family member with chronic illness, or helping their teen navigate a difficult time. You might find that time in nature also helps you connect with yourself and with other adults who might enjoy that same outdoor activity. Even if nothing particularly distressing is happening in your life, we encourage you to prioritize time outdoors, in nature, every week. If you're not able to schedule time outdoors with your child, still try to make time for it without guilt. Give yourself grace that you are doing the best you can and don't let perfect be the enemy of the improved. Then take a step back and think about some of the barriers you might be facing and how you might gradually overcome them. Remember, you are trying to do something that is good for your health, makes you a better parent, and allows you to model self-care to your child.

Cultivating a Family Connection to Nature

Cultivating a Family Connection to Nature

Do you consider yourself outdoorsy? We want to assure you that wherever you are on your journey to finding connection, meaning, and joy in the outdoors, there is a way for you to support your children in developing their relationship with nature. You may have grown up in a family that regularly hiked or camped; you have all the gear and feel confident exposing your children to outdoor adventures. Or you may have grown up in an urban area where neighborhood parks and school field trips were your main exposure to outdoor play. Perhaps you participated in a school environmental education program or a wilderness-based summer camp that was transformative. Maybe you grew up in a family where no one wanted to go camping in the wilderness, but your family loved picnics, barbeques, gardening, or walks.

Or you might be someone who does not consider themselves outdoorsy at all and is reluctant to spend time outdoors. You might feel daunted at the list (and cost!) of specialized gear that seems necessary for some outdoor activities. You may not want to spend hours away from electricity and plumbing or choose to sleep in a sleeping bag. We've come across patients, friends, and members of our own extended families who fit into each of these categories.

We also recognize that how we feel about the outdoors is influenced by our culture. And our culture is shaped by many things, including the neighborhood where we live, where we lived growing up, and the whole community that shares this space. Culture is also influenced by the ethnic or racial heritage of our ancestors, their experiences, and whether they were always here or whether they immigrated 2 centuries ago or 2 years ago. Probably most importantly, our culture is shaped most closely by our own family's priorities. Family shapes how you spend your time and what you decide to do together, and your family is your very first nature mentor. What we do in nature or in the time we offer our children in nature creates their culture. Since I (DG) grew up in western Washington, I was surprised to find that some families that had just moved to rainy Washington kept their children indoors during this weather even if they considered themselves outdoorsy. They brought their culture from their previous home, usually a warm, sunny climate, to the Pacific Northwest. In some cases, they did not even realize they had developed a bias for staying indoors during rain until it had been months of being inside. It became part of my routine to mention that families should encourage their kids to go out even in the rain. Although it took some convincing, I was able to help parents see that there were some real opportunities to play in the rain, so their children could learn about weather and how rain plays an important part in our ecosystem. Fortunately, how we express our culture is not fixed by our experiences growing up. We can borrow "nature culture" from one another, and we can share our nature culture with others to make outdoor play and exploration inviting for all children and their families.

REFLECTION: Think of how your family's culture has influenced your ideas and activities related to the outdoors and nature. What are some ways your culture has made it easier to be in nature? What are some of your cultural ways, beliefs, or fears that have held you or your children back from nature time? How have those factors in turn shaped your decisions about nature contact for your children?

Growing Outdoors Builds Resilience

Parents often share with us their challenges in encouraging their child to go outside, and we try to help them problem-solve and strategize on how to overcome those barriers. Hopefully, you will find some information and strategies that help your family reap the benefits of nature time and nature connection.

Weather-related challenges

One of the most common barriers families mention about spending time outdoors is the weather. Depending on where you live, there are probably times in the year when it's too hot, too cold, too wet… (basically, too unpleasant) to want to spend time outdoors. With cold temperatures and precipitation, you might be worried that your child will get sick from playing outdoors.

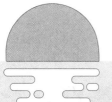

REFLECTION: What factors are in the way of you and/or your child spending more time outdoors?

Ask the Pediatrician

Q: We live in an area with rain (or snow) for many months of the year. Will my child get sick from being outside in wet weather?

A: This is such a common concern. But rest assured, only germs cause illness. As long as your child stays warm and mostly dry, it is fine for them to be in the rain. Use waterproof jackets or ponchos or hats or have them play under a covered area and check to make sure your child is staying warm. You can shorten the time you spend outdoors if it is very cold or wet.

With extreme heat, you might be concerned about sunburn, dehydration, or heat exhaustion. It's great to think about how to best prepare for the weather, but try not to let the weather stop your family from getting outdoors. Growing up in the Pacific Northwest, our children got used to hiking, biking, and playing through some drizzle. There's even a claim, perhaps an urban legend, that Seattle has the most per-capita sales of sunglasses in the United States—because we keep losing our sunglasses in the long stretches without sunshine! While we can attest to glorious, sunny summers, our families knew to dress in layers, have our fleece hoodies nearby, and invest in shoes that would keep our feet dry.

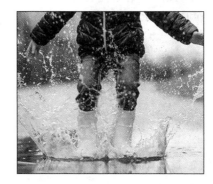

Of course, playing outside during a light rain shower can be fun, but when lightning, hail, or other dangerous weather appears, it's best to go inside during a storm. You may need to modify how long your child stays out-

doors if it is very hot or very cold. On extremely hot days, avoid scheduling outdoor activities from late morning to midafternoon, when the sun is the strongest, and take breaks in the shade to reapply sunscreen and hydrate. These are great opportunities to teach your child about how they can be ready for differ-ent weather conditions by learning to be flexible if conditions change. The first few times my (PT) son's soccer practice got canceled for lightning or smoky

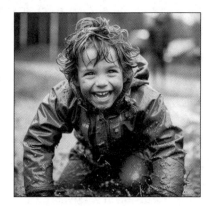

conditions from nearby wildfires in the summer, he was disappointed. It gave us an opportunity to talk about the reasons why practice got canceled and how to be safe in those circumstances. It is good to remember, though, that except for the most extreme weather conditions, it is safe for most children to be outdoors if they are dressed appropriately and prepared. In fact, play-ing in the rain can be fun! There's a German saying, "Du bist doch nicht aus Zucker!" or "You're not made of sugar!" implying that you won't melt, so go ahead and enjoy the rain.

One additional benefit of having your child spend some time outdoors in less ideal weather is that it helps them learn how to be prepared for different con-ditions and be resilient to things like heat, cold, wind, and rain. You can talk with your child about how they react when unexpected weather changes their plans or when their socks get wet. They can also learn the consequences of not wearing the right gear, which will likely prepare them better for the next

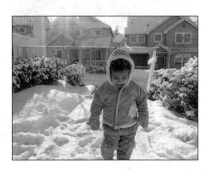

time! Even toddlers and preschoolers can learn how to dress for the weather so they are comfortable outdoors. Have fun with it! Teach your child to look at the weather forecast and plan their outfits and outdoor activities accordingly. Use these weather opportunities as a chance to talk about weather and climate, including why we need precipitation

Nature Nugget: No Such Thing as Bad Weather

We are inspired by a famous Scandinavian saying: *There's no such thing as bad weather, only bad clothing.* Here are some suggestions for keeping your child comfortable and safe in different weather conditions.

Cold weather: Dress in layers of synthetic or wool clothes, avoid cotton clothing, and remember to have a hat, gloves, and warm socks.

Wet weather: Dress in quick-dry and/or waterproof clothing, and remember to have waterproof shoes/boots so their feet stay dry (or keep extra socks on hand); full-body waterproof suits work well for young children to play outdoors in wet conditions.

Hot weather: Dress in breathable, loose, light-colored fabrics like cotton or linen, and consider having a hat and other clothing to protect from the sun.

Sun exposure: Time outdoors is the best way for you and your child to get some important vitamin D, and you can take some steps to make sure all of you are protected from the sun's powerful rays. Also, remember that sunburn can happen even on cloudy or cool days. To protect their skin, keep children in the shade and encourage wearing wide-brimmed hats, sunglasses, and clothes that cover children's arms and legs. For children older than 6 months, use sunscreen with an SPF of 15 or higher on any exposed skin. Apply sunscreen 30 minutes before outdoor time and reapply it at least every 2 hours—or more often if children are sweating or spending time in the water.

and water. Highlight the possibilities of playing and learning in these weather conditions, whether playing (safely) in the rain, splashing in puddles, checking out worms, or catching rain in a container. If it snows near you, help your child get excited and prepared for measuring inches of snowfall, building snowmen, and finding places for sledding and other snow play.

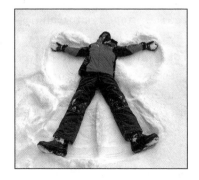

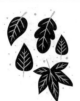

When Great Grandma Was a Baby

I collect vintage and antique parenting books. I think it is fascinating how previous generations raised children, and I like to learn what the cultural norms were for a certain time. In a booklet for parents from 1909, taking your infant outside every day is prescribed from birth. The expert author reports that this "daily airing" is important for good health, vigor, and the proper development of the lungs.

—Danette

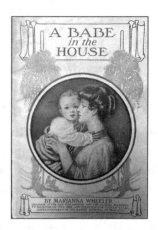

And honestly, many children are perfectly fine to continue playing outdoors even when the adults with them are feeling deterred by the weather. But even the least ideal weather conditions can create fun memories, so get out there with your kids!

Safety concerns

We know that parents worry about their child's safety at any age and sometimes must make difficult decisions as they think about how to prioritize safety against other parenting goals. As pediatricians, we are also always thinking about what guidance we can give families and our young patients about balancing harm prevention and health promotion. When children run and jump and climb, as they might when they play outdoors, there is certainly some risk for injuries. Outdoor activities around water or at varying heights or in more remote areas come with risks. However, when children experience new challenges, take some risks, solve problems, and achieve milestones, they often gain confidence and become better prepared to handle themselves in the future.

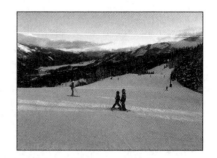

My husband and I (PT) are reluctant skiers; not having grown up skiing, we never got very comfortable with this activity. We initially delayed any sort of ski lessons for our children, as it sounded like too much work, too much gear, and too much risk to take on in order to tow little ones to an activity where everyone spends a day in the cold. Over time, we were convinced by some friends that starting the process for our children when they were young and when their friends were learning might actually be a good idea so they achieved the skills and confidence needed and didn't end up feeling like us as adults! So, with lots of guidance from experienced friends, we signed up our children for ski lessons and they've both gone on to become avid expert skiers who can confidently navigate the mountains and enjoy this fun wintertime activity. We opted for lessons over several years to make sure they learned proper techniques and were supervised on the slopes until they were older. Once they surpassed our ski skill level, my husband and I decided to "retire" from this sport and have found that we love cross-country skiing and snowshoeing instead.

As parents, it is important to consider what level of risk you are comfortable with for your child and take steps to ensure they are engaging in age-appropriate activities, using recommended gear, and experiencing a safe

Ask the Pediatrician

Q: I don't have great rain or snow clothes for my child (or myself). How can I get these kinds of clothes at low or no cost?

A: Check local thrift shops and back-to-school drives in your community for low-cost items. Another idea is checking with your place of worship or a nonprofit for a clothes drive. Depending on where you live, your local Buy Nothing, thrift store, Freecycle, or Goodwill may have gently used clothes in addition to equipment. Don't forget to check with family and friends for hand-me-downs. Social media sites like Facebook Marketplace and Nextdoor also have pages that list items for free. Make sure that any used clothing or equipment is in good condition and of the correct size to keep you or your child well protected. Preschools and schools may also have programs where you can find, borrow, or purchase jackets and other gear at lower costs.

Continued on the next page

? Ask the Pediatrician (*continued*)

Q: I did not grow up doing many outdoor activities, and I have never been camping. But now my child wants to go on a school camping trip, and I'm worried about their safety. Should I let them go?

A: It can feel scary to let your child do something that even you have not experienced. Have an open conversation with your child about their understanding of what is involved and how they will prepare for this trip. Share your concerns and ask questions. Ask to speak with the adult(s) who will be attending and supervising the trip. Ask them questions about things you are concerned about (eg, sleeping arrangements, weather, safety from others, safety from animals), and relay any of your child's health conditions or diet restrictions. If possible, check with the parents of other children who are participating to see how they feel. Balance the risks of letting your child go with what they may gain from this experience: knowledge, responsibility, appreciation for things they may otherwise take for granted, time away from screens, and an opportunity for growth and outdoor learning. Ultimately, you will need to feel comfortable with the information you receive before letting them go.

environment. Children or parents who have mobility limitations or other health concerns may need to be extra cognizant of safety considerations (see Chapter 4 for more on this topic). Some parents may not be familiar with the outdoor activities that their child's peers are doing or their child is asking to do, so their concerns are understandable. It can be helpful to seek out classes or camps or enlist the support of other trusted, experienced adults to help you navigate new territories regarding outdoor activities with your child.

Each family has a different threshold for when they might feel comfortable with their child spending time outdoors without adult supervision. Depending on various factors such as their age and personality and your neighborhood, it's up to you to decide when you feel it will be OK to let them spend some time outdoors alone or with peers. You can provide guidance on how far they can venture and how often they should check in with you. Discuss what steps to take and how to find adults they can ask if they need help. Have a conversation with your child to discuss both your comfort level and theirs as you give them more independence, and begin by taking small steps. You might have them start by checking the mail by themselves or visiting a nearby neighbor's house before expanding their "roaming distance" to a larger area. For older children, you can establish rules about calling or messaging you once they reach a destination, or at regular intervals, or if they are running late coming home. There are even templates online for teen behavior contracts that parents and teens can use to discuss and agree on rules regarding where they are allowed to go, curfews, and consequences.

Water safety

Engaging in activities in or near water can be tremendous fun for families and children of all ages, but it is important to follow some precautions to ensure safety. My husband and I (PT) had a scare with my younger son at the beach one day when he was about 2 years old. It was probably a matter of less than 5 minutes that felt like an eternity when, as a result of a miscommunication, my husband and I each thought the other was watching our son. We panicked, ran around the beach looking for him, and alerted the lifeguard through tears. It turned out that he had overshot where we were sitting with our beach blanket and had gotten engrossed in a digging adventure a little farther behind us. We of course had assumed the worst and focused our search close to the water. That evening, we bought a life jacket and vowed that he would have to wear it at all times near the water even if there were no plans for him to go into the water. We also made it a priority for our children to learn swimming early.

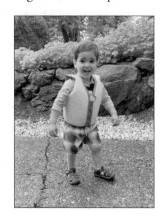

Learning to swim is so important, and most children are ready to learn by their fourth birthday, if not earlier. Look into swimming lessons offered locally and continue them until your child is a comfortable, strong swimmer. When at a swimming pool, near or in open water, or at a water park, always ensure there is adult supervision within arm's reach of a young child or inexperienced swimmer. For many families, fishing is a tradition that brings generations together, so children often get involved at a young age. Remember, young children will need close supervision near water even if swimming is not part of the plan. Always swim with others and set water safety rules with your child. Even if you or your child knows how to swim, always have your child wear an appropriately sized, buckled-up US Coast Guard–approved life jacket or life vest when swimming in open water (eg, lake, river, ocean, swimming pool) or when on a boat, an inner tube, a paddleboard, or the dock. You may need to remind your older children of water safety and communicate your rules to other adults supervising your children near water when you are not there. We recommend that parents and other adults who spend time with their child take a cardiopulmonary resuscitation (CPR) course to be better prepared to handle any emergencies. Check if the American Red Cross, your community hospitals, or other local organizations offer CPR classes near you, or you can use the helpful Find a Class tool through the American Red Cross website (www.redcross.org/take-a-class/cpr/cpr-training). HealthyChildren.org also has many resources for families about water safety, including drowning prevention (www.healthychildren.org/English/safety-prevention/at-play/Pages/Water-Safety-And-Young-Children.aspx).

Safety gear

Ensure that you and your children always wear activity-appropriate gear for activities such as bicycling, snow sports, ice-skating, team sports, and equestrian sports. There are differences between helmet types, so make sure you are using the correct helmet type for the activity. Encourage your child to use a helmet by letting them choose one they like and/or letting them decorate it. It is important to note that helmets need to be replaced if they are involved in a crash or become damaged or outgrown. It's best to avoid using previously owned helmets, if possible. Other sports may have special protective gear that is recommended by your child's team or coach.

If your family hunts or fishes, you may have guns and knives in your home. Children are naturally curious about these powerful tools. Safety training is mandatory, but even if they can show and tell you the safety rules, you must keep these items locked up. Hiding them is not enough. The American Academy of Pediatrics recommends firearms be kept in a lockbox or safe, unloaded, with the ammunition stored separately. See HealthyChildren.org (www.healthychildren.org/English/safety-prevention/at-home/Pages/Handguns-in-the-Home.aspx) for more information on safety guidelines.

Insects and animal safety

Being in nature often means we might encounter insects or creatures. While playing outdoors, children could encounter stray or wild animals. You can take steps to keep your child safe and healthy. Choose areas where children can be safe from snakes, rodents, and other animals that may be hazardous by noting any posted warnings, staying on populated trails, and learning how to respond if you do encounter different creatures. I (PT) remember that before a family trip to Glacier National Park in Montana, we became keenly aware of the risk for bear encounters there. We brought bear spray, were alert to posted warnings about animals, stayed in groups during our hike, and had our kids watch online videos about what to do if you come upon a bear. For some families, it may be best to choose guided activities in wilderness areas.

Outdoor activities can also increase the risk for bugbites. Some children experience significant local reactions with red, swollen, itchy areas developing around the insect bite. Bugs, including mosquitoes, ticks, fleas, and flies, can also spread germs. For times when you know you will be around bugs, dress children in clothing that covers their arms and legs, and cover strollers and baby carriers with mosquito netting. Be aware of ticks in areas where they might be present, such as forests, tall grasses, and brush, and check clothing and gear for ticks frequently. Tuck your child's pants into their socks for extra protection. You can also use insect repellents on infants and children older than 2 months. DEET-containing repellents that contain no more than 30% DEET for children are one of the most effective insect repellents. Repellants should be applied on top of sunscreen and with supervision of younger children.

We want you to feel confident when sending your children outside where there might be pests like ticks. Only use products with proven effectiveness and as directed. Ticks are rare in western Washington, and ticks that carry diseases are even more rare, so my family (DG) usually did not encounter them. But on a hike through a forest in the Midwest, my family and I were prepared with long sleeves, pants tucked in, and DEET sprayed onto our clothes. Even so, my daughter and I both had ticks in our hair attached at the nape of our necks. This was scary for all of us, but only because we were not used to dealing with ticks. Knowing what to do and how to remove them put us at ease, so we were able to enjoy the rest of the hike. Be sure to check your child over completely, even with the usual precautions in place, after outdoor time in areas with ticks. You can learn more about removing ticks at HealthyChildren.org (www.healthychildren.org/English/health-issues/conditions/from-insects-animals/Pages/how-to-remove-a-tick.aspx).

Plant safety

It could be an interesting and fun activity to learn about different types of plants. Show your child pictures and descriptions online or from a book and then look for them outdoors. A favorite late summer activity for my family (PT) has been picking wild blackberries! We've talked about and looked at pictures of different berries and identified blackberries as safe to eat. We've taught our kids how to be careful about thorns and critters or bugs that may be nearby. You can teach your child how it's OK to look at these plants but not safe to touch or eat them unless they check with an adult first. Let your children know they should avoid touching and eating any plants that are unfamiliar to them. From a young age, your children can start to learn features of plants that could be harmful, like thorns or other sharp features and bark that could cause splinters. Show them pictures of poison ivy and poison oak and help them identify those plants that could give them an itchy rash if they come in contact with them. Many plants, wild berries, and mushrooms are also poisonous if eaten. Another idea is to plant a garden or even some seeds in a pot to learn about plants or fruit that are safe to touch or eat.

Air quality

Children are more sensitive than adults to health effects from breathing in polluted air, and their respiratory system is still developing until about age 21 years. Children with health conditions (including asthma and other lung diseases) have an even greater risk of becoming sick when the air quality is poor. Especially if you live in a region that is prone to air pollution or wildfire smoke, we recommend that you check the Air Quality Index (AQI) in your area before you or your family members spend time outdoors. The AQI is a useful tool to check local air quality and can be found online or in weather apps or the local newspaper. The AQI is measured from a range

Ask the Pediatrician

Q: I have heard that we shouldn't be outside when the air quality is bad, but I don't know how to find this out.

A: Since climate change is causing more extreme events such as wildfires, this can lead to the air pollution being significant in some areas; thus, there may be days that it is not safe for your child to explore nature outside. Check the government-maintained and frequently updated website AirNow (www.airnow.gov). Just enter your zip code or city and state. Children should not be active outside if the Air Quality Index is more than 100.

between 0 and 500, with a value of 50 or below representing good air quality, values above 100 being unhealthy for certain sensitive groups including all children, and values beyond that being unhealthy for all people (as the AQI gets higher). It is recommended that children not be active outside when the AQI is above 100 or in the orange, red, purple, or maroon zones (third, fourth, fifth, or sixth rows of Figure 3.1). In the Pacific Northwest, we are used to hearing from schools, sports, and other outdoor activity leaders when children's outdoor times need to be modified because the AQI is high from nearby wildfire smoke in the summers. As pediatricians, we especially recommend that our patients with asthma check AQIs during these times. I (DG) once had a patient who needed to be hospitalized for severe asthma after continuing to play soccer during wildfire smoke. It is relatively a newer development to have to consider air quality before going outside. Your parents likely did not think about this before you played outside when you were younger. But air quality in many places is often compromised. Figure 3.1 highlights the various activities children participate in and the recommended levels of air quality for such activities.

Figure 3.1. The Air Quality Guide for Particle Pollution

Air Quality Index	Who Needs to be Concerned?	What Should I Do?
Good 0-50		It's a great day to be active outside.
Moderate 51-100	Some people who may be unusually sensitive to particle pollution.	Unusually sensitive people: *Consider reducing* prolonged or heavy exertion. Watch for symptoms such as coughing or shortness of breath. These are signs to take it easier.
		Everyone else: It's a good day to be active outside.
Unhealthy for Sensitive Groups 101-150	Sensitive groups include people with heart or lung disease, older adults, children and teenagers.	Sensitive groups: *Reduce* prolonged or heavy exertion. It's OK to be active outside, but take more breaks and do less intense activities. Watch for symptoms such as coughing or shortness of breath.
		People with asthma should follow their asthma action plans and keep quick relief medicine handy.
		If you have heart disease: Symptoms such as palpitations, shortness of breath, or unusual fatigue may indicate a serious problem. If you have any of these, contact your health care provider.
Unhealthy 151 to 200	Everyone	Sensitive groups: *Avoid* prolonged or heavy exertion. Move activities indoors or reschedule to a time when the air quality is better.
		Everyone else: *Reduce* prolonged or heavy exertion. Take more breaks during all outdoor activities.
Very Unhealthy 201-300	Everyone	Sensitive groups: *Avoid all* physical activity outdoors. Move activities indoors or reschedule to a time when air quality is better.
		Everyone else: *Avoid* prolonged or heavy exertion. Consider moving activities indoors or rescheduling to a time when air quality is better.
Hazardous 301-500	Everyone	Everyone: *Avoid all* physical activity outdoors.
		Sensitive groups: Remain indoors and keep activity levels low. Follow tips for keeping particle levels low indoors.

Source: US Environmental Protection Agency. https://www.epa.gov/sites/default/files/2014-09/aqiguidepm.png. Accessed June 4, 2024.

Illnesses and the outdoors

Playing outdoors is often blamed for making children catch a cold or flu. Especially if you have family members who grew up in warmer climates, it can be difficult to convince them that it's OK for children to play outdoors in the cold. In our office, we see plenty of over-bundled little ones because their parents or grandparents are worried about them getting sick. While we agree that children need to be appropriately dressed for the weather, remember that viruses that cause colds and flu spread and circulate more between people indoors. We learned during the COVID-19 pandemic that outdoor spaces were safer than indoors for viral transmission, and this is true for other viruses and bacteria too. If your child is sick with a mild illness and feels up for spending some time outdoors, even on a porch or in a backyard, you might find that the change of scenery from the indoors, perhaps some sunshine, lifts their spirits and helps them feel better. For someone facing a long-term illness, there can also be benefits to spending time in or even looking at natural scenery. Studies have even shown that window views of nature or plants inside hospital rooms can support recovery from illness or surgery.

Navigating limited free time

You might be feeling like you'd love to get your child outdoors more but there just isn't enough time in the day or week to manage it all. Like many families, you are juggling jobs, school, activities, and other priorities. It may feel frustrating to hear all these wonderful benefits for having your child spend time in nature but not be able to do it all. Don't worry! Hopefully, some of our suggestions don't add to your list of to-dos but rather give you an opportunity for some moments of joy or respite from the daily grind.

Bring current activities outdoors

One strategy is to think about events or activities that you or your child already do, together or separately, and see if you could move any of the indoor ones to outdoors. It may not be possible every day or even more than once a week, but finding even 30 minutes once a week and trying to make it happen regularly is better than no time outside. Most children benefit from routines, and if you can carve that out as special time with your child weekly, you might both look forward to it. Consider the following ideas:

- Bring homework or reading outdoors to a porch, a backyard, or, if you have access, a nearby park with a picnic bench. Even a window view of nature would be nice while reading or studying if the weather is not suitable for being outdoors.

Ask the Pediatrician

Q: We have a very athletic child, usually involved in 2 sports per season. Because of that, practices and games take up a lot of their time after school. How can we squeeze in nature time?

A: Many families struggle with overcommitment to sports. There are other pursuits that can swallow a disproportionate amount of your child's time, such as music, drama, or even academic pressures. We challenge you to step back and ask some hard questions.

- Are year-round sports (multiple sports or multiple teams for the same sport) affecting your child's sleep? Time spent with family or friends? Their opportunity to learn something new? Their overall health and/or happiness?

- Is the stress from coordinating this activity worth compromising all your child's (and usually family's) downtime, nature time, hobby time, or family mealtime?

Talk with your child and guide them in deciding what would make them happiest, even if that's reducing their sports commitments to balance their life. This difficult process is a very important teachable moment for growing your child's responsible decision-making. Even if you decide to stick with the high sports commitment, we encourage you to carve out some unstructured family time outdoors on a regular basis.

- Plan outdoor playdates, gatherings with friends or family, or celebrations. You might enjoy chatting with other adults at the park while your preschooler or elementary-aged child plays nearby. Picnics and potlucks and barbeques are wonderful ways to get the whole family outdoors! During the pandemic, our family (PT) did several campfire meetups even in the winter with everyone bundled up and enjoying warm cider.

- Go outdoors after it's dark if you feel comfortable doing so. This is a good option especially during the fall and winter, when the daylight hours are short. Dress warmly, bring a headlamp or flashlight, and take a walk or gaze at the night sky.

- If you have a dog, set some times for when you walk your dog together with your child.
- If you pick up your child from school, linger a little longer on the schoolyard, if that's allowed. Ask if the schoolyard is available on weeknights or weekends for community use.
- Schedule a Saturday morning visit to the park with a younger child or Sunday afternoon walk together with your family. Consider including grandparents or other friends or relatives.

Connecting in Nature While Social Distancing

We all had to learn new ways to do old things during the COVID-19 pandemic. Children attended school remotely, families celebrated milestones virtually, and people of all ages donned masks and navigated social distancing. So much of what we did felt unnatural and bizarre (think of when you were isolating from family members in the same home or not hugging people you love). One hopeful trend that emerged was the recognition that being outdoors was safer than indoors for preventing infection. Heeding public health guidance, many people started feeling more comfortable returning to restaurants if they could sit outdoors and organizing social gatherings in backyards, patios, and parks.

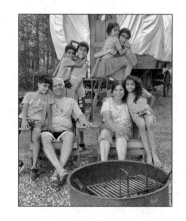

My parents were in their 70s the first time they went camping (it was actually glamping, but close enough). In the summer of 2021, the first time I saw my parents after 18 months was when I ran out of our car and hugged them in a campground in Maine. It was the safest way my family felt comfortable meeting up with 8 adults and 6 children coming from cities across the country. From birthday parties to weddings, from playdates to family reunions, it became clear that it was possible to gather, celebrate, and dine together outdoors. We hope many people continue to choose the outdoors for these events and more.

—Pooja

If you have plants growing inside, start some outdoors in pots or in your yard. Some neighborhoods have community gardens where you can get a patch if there is limited space around your home.

School and extracurriculars

Think about your child's current school and extracurricular activities that might already be giving your child opportunities to be in nature. Counting sports participation as outdoor time can be tricky depending on the sport and the setting. If your child is running on trails every day during cross-country team practice, they are likely getting a good dose of nature. Soccer practice in a field surrounded by buildings will be good more so as an opportunity for physical activity and team social skills development but less so as an opportunity for nature contact. So just keep that in mind as you think about how much cumulative nature your child is getting, and for those who are mostly doing sports, you might want to think about ways to enrich with other opportunities.

When your child has a vacation from school, especially during the summer, those breaks are wonderful opportunities to have them spend time in nature. When my children were younger, I (PT) usually needed child care for many weeks of the summer and my philosophy was that they should participate in activities they didn't typically get to do during the busy school year. With this idea in mind, they were exposed to a range of different outdoor-oriented camps—wilderness skills, parkour, kayaking/sailing, and more. I didn't realize we were starting a tradition that has lasted over a decade when we

discovered the camp at Shoofly Farm in Washington. This is a day camp where children get to care for bunnies, ride horses, make and churn butter, cook over the campfire, and explore the suburban farm. My children started there as camp-ers and loved it so much that they eventually became helpers and then assistant counselors. We have heard from others about them or their child having a long-term connection with a nature-based summer experience (day camps and over-night camps) and how foundational and memorable that has been for them.

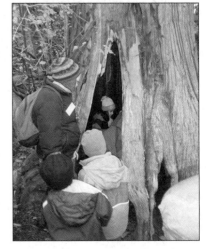

If this seems intriguing to you, explore what options are available by asking around and checking online. YMCAs across the country often run camps like these, and sometimes cultural organizations do too. Your child may enjoy the experience more if you coordinate going with their friends and may even discover a new passion.

Nature as Exercise

A friend's teenager who did not consider herself athletic was dreading the physical education (PE) requirement in high school. She had heard that students were required to do timed runs and send in videos of themselves doing assorted exercises, and all of that sounded dreadful. Her parents noticed the option for interested students to join a new hiking club at school that would give students PE credit and encouraged her to sign up. This was a turning point for their daughter. She looked forward to the twice-weekly hikes through this club. She made new friends as she chatted with them during their hikes in the woods near the high school. Much to her parents' surprise, she came home with lists of hikes she wanted to try with them on the weekends!

While PE should never feel dreadful or traumatic, this story was particularly heartwarming in that it awakened a connection with the outdoors in a teen who did not previously think of herself as having one. I've also learned that there are low-cost ways for children to try some outdoor activities that may seem inaccessible or costly, such as sailing, golf, and skiing. For example, Youth on Course (www.youthoncourse.org) is dedicated to making golf more accessible and gives youth access to thousands of golf courses around the country for only $5 each time. I know several teens, including my son, who have developed a passion for golf thanks to this program. Others lost interest in team sports as they got older but discovered a passion for these types of activities that can rekindle a love for the outdoors. With the right experience, it's never too late for an older child or adult to find a connection to the natural world.

—Pooja

Seek help from others

Also, consider whether someone from your "village" of family or friends could help take your child outdoors when you cannot, and then maybe you can return the favor another time. During summers, a few adults could take turns taking children from each other's families to a nearby park or lake. Additionally, remember to encourage the adults who care for your child on a regular basis (eg, grandparents, babysitters, child care providers, teachers) to find outdoor and nature-time opportunities for your child, since they may be spending more daytime hours with them than you.

Challenges in accessing nature

We recognize that not everyone has easy access to parks, greenspaces, and other types of nature contact in their communities. Even if there is a park nearby, you may not feel comfortable letting your child play there for various reasons, such as concerns about getting there safely, strangers, unsafe conditions, and more. It is important to mention that Black, Indigenous, People of Color (BIPOC) in the United States have not had the same opportunities to enjoy the outdoors for a variety of reasons, including systemic historical inequities in where parks were chosen to be built and feelings of safety in those spaces. In recent years, there has been an explosion of organizations and programs supporting diversity, inclusion, and belonging in the outdoors, including ones specifically focused on youth.

There are affinity organizations that are national or statewide in scope with local affiliates, or your city or community may have its own. Many specifically support children in their exploration of nature or have sections devoted to getting children out in nature. Some organizations are BIPOC led and devoted to people of a specific race or ethnic culture, encouraging and facilitating a wide variety of nature experiences. These affinity groups include Latino Outdoors, Black Girls Trekkin', Outdoor Asian, Unlikely Hikers, Black Outside, Outdoor Afro, The Bronze Chapter, and many others. Organizations such as Backyard Basecamp are also leading the way in increasing equitable access to nature. Founder and Executive Director Atiya Wells came across a 10-acre vacant property in her neighborhood in northeast Baltimore and led a land reclamation and environmental justice movement to create BLISS Meadows, which serves as a home for community dinners, environmental education, nature play spaces, and gardens. The Sierra Club features Inspiring Connections Outdoors groups all over the United States that host outdoor experiences, provide gear, and transport children who

Together in Nature

Those who think that nature is a place to immerse yourself in quiet solitude have not met some of my friends and family. Sure, there are moments of quiet reflection during a lull in conversation during a walk or as we eat a picnic dinner at sunset next to a lake. There may be peaceful moments sitting on a park bench and observing a nearby tree or bird. But for the most part, when my family or friends gather outdoors, it is vibrant and noisy. There is often food involved (which we keep safe from wild animals and dispose of properly). There is conversation and laughter as well as a sense of joy being outdoors together.

There are certainly individual, family, and cultural differences in how people interact with and enjoy the outdoors. Some may love solo hiking, using that time to reflect or just be present. Others show up in groups to a state park, prepared to cook meals and share stories around a campfire until the guilt of quiet hours compels us to call it a night. Especially as people of color, when we are in large groups in outdoor spaces, my friends and I have talked about feeling conscious about our presence. An important consideration is that Black and Brown people may feel unsafe in some outdoor spaces alone. Experiencing nature in groups is one strategy that can help alleviate that feeling.

—Pooja

don't have access to nature otherwise (www.sierraclub.org/ico). There are also affinity groups supporting LGBTQ+ families exploring nature. Look for these supportive groups near you. Some we are familiar with include Pride Outside, LGBT+ Outdoors, The Venture Out Project, and Brave Trails.

Also, look at your local zoo, parks and recreation, library, or cultural center for resources and group nature experiences. Some pediatricians and pediatric practices are also leading their patients and families on nature experiences with an emphasis on language or ethnic culture of the affinity group. The magic in these groups is how they are making the outdoors more accessible and comfortable through shared culture.

A related concept is known as *emotional safety*. Some individuals or families have had traumatic experiences accessing nature even in a greenspace

Action Item: Think of what factors are preventing your child and your family from accessing nature as much as you would like. Can you think of potential work-arounds to overcome some of those challenges? Try to apply at least one solution within the next week.

Ask the Pediatrician

Q: I am unsure if we have a safe park near where we live. What are some ways to find safe areas nearby?

A: Check for local, state, and national parks near you by using various park-finder websites.

- **NATIONAL PARK AND HISTORICAL SITES:** See Find a Park (www.nps.gov/findapark/index.htm) and Find Your Park (https://findyourpark.com).

- **STATE PARKS OR CITY PARKS:** Using an online search engine, type in your area or city (such as "Minnesota state parks" or "city of Chattanooga parks").

- **NATURAL AREAS:** Think beyond parks to other natural areas such as Heritage Trees (https://americanheritagetrees.org) and, of course, public schoolyards as well as outdoor areas around community centers and libraries.

Many of these public spaces have informal but engaging outdoor spaces that all are welcome to use. We often think of urban areas with limited park spaces, but sometimes the people in rural areas also lack nearby, safe outdoor places and face transportation barriers. All these inequities in access need to change. If you feel unsafe in a park near you, consider planning your outing to the park when there are official, planned activities or supervision. Many communities are increasing the use of parks by hosting activities or presentations and even supervision that make the area safer. Plus, going with others may help with some safety concerns. Another idea is to check if your child's preschool or school allows families to use their outdoor spaces during nonschool hours.

considered safe by standard definitions. Or they may have heard about an unsafe situation in nature and now are too fearful to be outside. It takes special planning and repeated reassurance to overcome those fears for those who do not feel emotionally safe outdoors. As a parent, listen to your child's fears and concerns. Take small steps over time to get back outdoors safely and comfortably. Affinity groups are meant to be emotionally supportive and may help mitigate fears after emotional trauma. Even short, nearby nature excursions in a group can help extend nature time. If repeated attempts in supportive groups do not begin to lessen the fear, a mental health professional may be able to help.

Defining *Outdoorsy* for Ourselves

As we mentioned at the beginning of this chapter, we recognize that being outdoors and outdoorsy can look different for each of us. So, if you appreciate the nature and health connection and want to give your child those opportunities but would prefer not to be going all in with wilderness experiences yourself, it is still possible to offer that to your child. Many communities have nature-based preschools as well as school- and community-based clubs and programs that will help your child spend lots of hours outdoors. Connect with friends or families that may already be doing an activity you want to try, and see if they can guide you or go with you. Perhaps you could visit the library and pick out books together that have nature-based themes as a way to have some shared nature experiences. Remember to use positive language that encourages children to be curious about nature and feel connected to the earth.

However, if you love being outdoors, but your child is the reluctant one, try to explore what it is that is holding them back. Are they worried about something that could be addressed by finding a different location or type of activity? Would they be more likely to spend time outdoors if they had friends with them? Could you start with more familiar spaces close to home or their school? For example, we know many families that have had children practice camping indoors or in a backyard tent before a real campground experience. Find out what your child finds fun and see what ways you can add nature to those activities.

Ask the Pediatrician

Q: I work 2 jobs and have a relative babysit my child. What nature exposure ideas are there for inside the apartment since I don't feel comfortable with them going outside?

A: Your child's caregiver can find many ways to instill nature and the environment into their daily activities. They can use the windows to point out nearby nature, such as flowers and trees or different types of rain clouds, to your child. Also, have indoor plants or flowers for your child to explore. Maybe they can plant something together with the caregiver and watch it grow over time. Learning about how food grows and exploring textures and tastes of fruits and vegetables are other ideas for indoor nature activities. Collect a box of items from your family nature walks and keep them for the caregiver to go through, create crafts, or make gifts for others with your child, using acorns, leaves, rocks, sticks, and other bits. Don't forget to ask your child's caregiver to read nature-themed books to your infant or toddler.

Q: My child has a tantrum every time we try to go back inside after being outdoors. I don't even want to go out anymore. What can we do?

A: This is a common problem, especially when your little one is having so much fun! As with everything, it is good to plan the time and the effort it will take for the transition from outdoors to indoors. Before you go out, remind your child that you will be spending 20 minutes outside. Give a 2-minute heads-up. Pack up any bags or equipment first, then shepherd your toddler toward your transportation or toward home. Be firm but unemotional. Sometimes the fun part of tantrums for toddlers is how emotional a parent can become. If you are in nature with others, it can be easier to leave if everyone goes at the same time, so maybe plan that in advance with the other adults. As children get older, they can begin to understand the concept of time and delayed gratification. If you think your child will understand that idea, you can have a fun treat or favorite activity ready for them when you get home. Talk about this treat/activity before you leave and remind them often while you are out. If you

Continued on the next page

Ask the Pediatrician (*continued*)

think the tantrums are happening because your child gets too hungry or it's close to mealtime when you are trying to leave, consider bringing a small snack with you to give them during outdoor time.

Q: My child just wants to hang out in their room and play computer games. How can I get my child outside more when they seem to have little to no interest?

A: First, have a real conversation with your child about moods. Is your child feeling depressed or anxious? Ask this using many different words (eg, "feeling low," "feeling bad," "feeling worried"). Make sure things are OK at school and with friends. Ask directly about bullying, either of them or other kids at school. Also, make sure your child is truly getting enough sleep; so many children use their phone for social media and online conversations when they should be sleeping. This should be avoided by making phones be put away at night or, if the child is not mature enough to do this on their own, turning off the internet or cellular connections. Finally, find out what computer game they are enjoying. Plan how they can blend this with nature time. The simplest is just taking the computer game outside. Maybe explore computer games or phone apps that have to be played outside. For teens who have social media access, consider having them create a social media page to post their regular nature photographs, whimsi- cal nature photographs, or outdoor action shots. Or they can create a slideshow or album to share with friends and family. Maybe you can brainstorm new hobbies like cooking (eg, learn foraging, start gardening), biking, orienteering, or geocaching. See if they're willing to go outside with a friend or groups of friends. Suggest signing them up with their friends for a structured after-school or summer oppor- tunity that will provide nature time. If none of these ideas work, or if you find out your child has had some troubling moods, consult your child's pediatrician.

Nature Nugget: Nature Mentors and Allies

Nature mentors are experienced guides who can support others in experiencing the outdoors through actions such as providing encouragement, giving advice, lending gear, and, perhaps, accompanying them on a new adventure. *Nature allies* are reliable supporters who make it more likely that both of you will get outdoors and have a great time.

As someone who did not grow up doing many adventurous outdoor activities, I (PT) truly recognize the value of nature mentors and allies in my life. I am grateful to have had confident, experienced guides who nudged, supported, and encouraged outdoor activities that seemed daunting. As a child, I tried downhill skiing once when some family friends invited us to join them on a ski weekend trip. Since my parents were recent immigrants from India with many other priorities as they raised 3 children in a new country, it would have been highly unlikely for them to have planned that trip alone. Plus, none of us owned ski pants or jackets! The friends who invited us not only arranged ski gear but, importantly, provided both the vision and the support to make it happen.

Make it a goal to be your child's first nature mentor and nature ally! And it's great to think of other people, like family members, child care providers, and friends, who can also serve as nature mentors and nature allies for you and your child to spend time outdoors, perhaps by trying new activities. You never know what you might be able to achieve and enjoy. Also, think of ways you could be a nature mentor or nature ally for another family or your children's friends.

Each of Us Belongs in Nature

We encourage you to explore and find some outdoor activity that you and your child are willing to try together. From a young age, children listen to and watch their adult caregivers, and what you model for them is critical. Sharing nature experiences is a powerful way for families to connect with each other, create positive memories, and build a foundation for health and well-being. Each of us has our own history of personal, family, and community experiences related to the outdoors that likely influence how we think about spending time in nature today. We believe that each of us belongs in nature and encourage you to explore what that looks like for you and your family.

Navigating Nature for Children With Special Health Care Needs

Navigating Nature for Children With Special Health Care Needs

$\mathcal{A}$s much as we would love every child to have unbridled opportunities to be in nature, we have seen many patients who face challenges or restrictions to engaging in outdoor nature-based activities because of a medical condition. Children with special health care needs or certain conditions may require modifications and additional considerations when planning time in nature. Many of our outdoor spaces are not set up for accessibility for those with disabilities or movement restrictions compared to those without. Even if your child hasn't been specifically diagnosed with a disability or chronic condition, they may experience the world a bit differently than other children, or be delayed in their development, or have a temporary condition that will make nature experiences more difficult. Sometimes, there must be accommodations in nature because a child needs their activities to be restricted in order to manage their medical condition. And sometimes it is the parents or caregivers who may have conditions that affect their ability to get outdoors. When seeking out nature-rich outdoor spaces for a child with special health care needs, finding accessible design that is engaging for *all* children, together at the same time, can be a challenge. It can feel discouraging or overwhelming to create nature opportunities when children or adults face accessibility challenges.

REFLECTION: Does anyone in your family or friend group have a medical condition or face an illness or injury that makes it more challenging for them to spend time outdoors in nature? Are there steps you could take to help make nature contact easier for them?

In our pediatric practices, we make a point of helping families find the right accommodation or greenspace so all our patients and their families can spend time in nature together.

We have collected anecdotes and information from our experiences caring for families of children with special health care needs and share them as examples of how children facing various circumstances can and should glean the benefits of time in nature. Our list is not exhaustive. It consists of some accommodations and programs we have suggested for our patient's families or ideas we have learned about in caring for children with special health care needs. In our practices, these were the most common access and functional needs we saw in our patients. Your own experience and certainly the resources for children with special health care needs in your nearby area will be unique. Your child's health care practitioner can help you with specific considerations for your child and family; be sure to discuss this topic with them if it has not come up yet. They may also know about special programs, summer camps, or other experiences that are especially designed for children with special health care needs near you. Even if your child does not have a condition that affects them when outside, you might find something here that resonates for your child or another person in your life.

For children with conditions that require special considerations in nature, make sure that the needs are clearly documented and readily available for outings. This is especially important at child care, school, and any activities when a parent or caregiver is not immediately available. You can find examples of these health plans or emergency information forms online, not only for health care (www.acep.org/by-medical-focus/pediatrics/medical-forms/emergency-information-form-for-children-with-special-health-care-needs) but also for child care (https://nrckids.org/files/appendix/AppendixO(2019).pdf).

Considerations for People With Mobility Challenges

Many children with difficulty moving, such as those with weakness or extreme stiffness in their legs (eg, caused by cerebral palsy, some metabolic conditions or dystrophies, or significant developmental delay), children with limb shortening (short stature or dwarfism), or children who use a wheelchair, crutches, or walkers, can have a much harder time getting out in nature. Uneven terrain, sandy or soft soil, and snow and ice make it important for families to consider how they will experience nature time. Yet research shows that nature and nature-related activities are potentially even more important for these children, as nature time improves physical, mental, and social health.

For these children, the physical barriers to getting outside can be overcome with planning and accommodation. Fortunately, more and more communities are building playgrounds, park and beach access, and trails that are safe for people in wheelchairs and with unsteady gait. But your child may also feel reluctant to enter outdoor spaces that are physically accessible if they don't

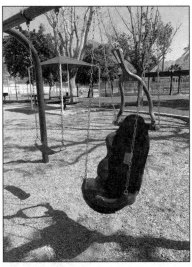

Adaptive swing for an older child needing support.

feel confident about their skills or are worried about feeling welcome there.

Nature Nugget: Eli's Park Project

Eli's Park Project in Seattle, WA, was inspired by a boy, Eli, who was born with Down syndrome. Through an inspiring community-engaged design process and fundraising effort, this group supported the construction of Pathways Park, an inclusive, nature-based park that will be both physically and socially accessible. Check out the website (www.elispark.org) for more information.

Since 2012, the concept of "accessible design" has been supported through the Americans with Disabilities Act standards that require playground equipment and facilities to have an accessible pathway to the edge of a play area. This is a start, but accessible design needs to consider blending the needs of all children together and to not simply address access for those with mobility challenges. Maybe there is a way for you to contribute to improved accessible design at a local park in your community and turn your park into one with "universal design." This would add features that allow all people of differing abilities, size, and confidence to engage with all their senses in the greenspace together.

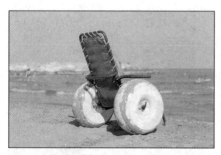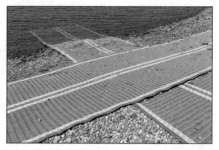

Beach wheelchairs and mobility mats may be available at some local parks.

Explore community programs that support inclusive and supportive outdoor programming for children of all abilities. You could work with a physical therapist, recreational therapist, or other professionals involved in your child's care to find ways to best support your child in comfortably experiencing nature. We also suggest checking with your local Family Voices group (https://familyvoices.org) and Easterseals (www.easterseals.com/our-programs/camping-recreation/recreation-and-sports.html) for more ideas.

Some community groups and nonprofit organizations are also funding adaptive equipment that can be lent to community members to make nature experiences accessible. We suggest families start by checking the parks that are nearby. National, state, and local parks often have websites with details about accommodation for those with physical challenges. The Americans with Disabilities Act and other laws require that federally funded parks be accessible. Look online for trails that have been paved or made with a level boardwalk. Specifically for federal recreation sites, look into the America the Beautiful access pass for discounts on entering or for some activities within these federal greenspaces and parks (www.nps.gov/planyourvisit/passes.htm). For beach access, look to see if the park lends beach wheelchairs to patrons or has wheelchair access mats (ie, sturdy rubber mats that allow a wheelchair to roll onto a beach without sinking into the sand).

For snow and ski access, check online for accommodations provided by the park administration, by a community group, or by the business running the snow/ski park. Some of these groups lend the equipment you will need to experience nature, but sometimes they also coordinate and actually provide the nature activity. It can be very expensive to purchase adaptive equipment for those with these conditions, so finding the programs that lend items or coordinate outings will be helpful.

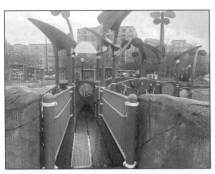 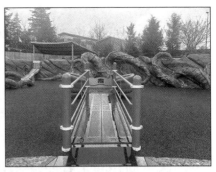

Inspiration Playground in Bellevue, WA, features equipment accessible to all, including children who use mobility assistant devices such as wheelchairs and walkers.

If you have the energy, your knowledge about what your child needs to fully experience a natural space is invaluable to community groups, and by 2025, there will be federal funding for states to provide this access through the Outdoors for All Act. Don't forget to ask your child's health care team, including physical therapists, recreational therapists, and equipment technicians, for their advice. They can offer all kinds of suggestions for your child and may know of groups trying to create more experiences for children with physical disabilities. Many of the suggestions previously mentioned will also be relevant if there are any adults in your family or social group who have mobility restrictions, so they, too, can be included.

Nature for Children With Breathing Issues

Some children have conditions that make it difficult to breathe when they are active or outside. This category might include asthma or other lung conditions, congenital heart disease, environmental allergies, and conditions requiring children to use ventilators or other forms of noninvasive ventilation. Some children who have been inactive can be so weak that they have trouble breathing when playing outside just from lack of conditioning. In most of these cases, we still want these children to be active, we still want them to be outside, and we still want them to experience nature. Physical activity can help with lung health and can actually help people with asthma and other heart and lung conditions stay healthier. Because children continue to grow new lung tissue into their early 20s, keep encouraging more and more activity outside—you might be surprised by your child not being as limited by their condition over time.

Nature Nugget: Disability-Focused Nonprofits

Whether you have internet at home or can access internet at a local library, we encourage you to look online for your local resources. They are abundant, and a quick search can help you find what your child or family needs. If internet searches are daunting, ask your local librarian to help you search your local area. Some examples include the following:

- Outdoors for All Foundation is a Pacific Northwest organization helping children with mobility issues experience nature (https://outdoorsforall.org).

- Environmental Traveling Companions also helps people with mobility disabilities experience nature, in northern California (https://etctrips.org).

- Open the Outdoors is a collection of resources for people with disabilities to enjoy outdoor recreation throughout Wisconsin (https://dnr.wisconsin.gov/topic/OpenOutdoors).

- Wilderness on Wheels is a Colorado-based organization helping people with mobility aids or limited mobility (www.wildernessonwheels.org).

- Disabilityinfo.org is a website created in Massachusetts for those who are disabled. The website includes not only a section to connect to nonprofits but also state and regional resources across the United States.

These are just a tiny fraction of the community-based nonprofits making nature accessible for those with mobility disabilities, including those with mobility aids. If you cannot find one near you, contact your state agency for children with special health care needs and ask for their recommendations.

Lung-related issues

For asthma and environmental allergies, the most important thing you can do is work with your child's health care practitioner to prevent symptoms. Sometimes we find that parents are reluctant to use preventive medications every day, but this daily use is the most important part of managing significant asthma and allergies. Let your child's doctor know if their physical activity is restricted. There are preventive medications for allergies and asthma, and if the first regimen tried does not allow your child to play and explore freely outside, go back and try others. We know you may hesitate to have many follow-up appointments with your child's pediatrician, but they truly want to find the right combination of medications to keep your child playing and active.

Sometimes asthma symptoms can be triggered by circumstances outdoors, like cold weather, pollen, or poor air quality, so extra precautions might be needed. If cold air is a trigger, your child could try covering their nose and mouth with a scarf or neck gaiter when outdoors. For environmental allergens, monitor pollen levels online (check out Pollen.com or most weather apps), have your child take a shower after playing outdoors, or avoid certain exposures that are typically problematic for them. Keeping their bedroom windows closed during high pollen counts can also help. If you live in an area where wildfire smoke or other pollutants are present, check the Air Quality Index to decide whether it is safe for your child to be outdoors on that day, but make it a priority to be out when the air is safe and clear (for more on this topic, see Air Quality in Chapter 3).

For children who use ventilators or noninvasive ventilation, outdoor time may be possible with machines that are portable and have batteries. It is always a good idea to have backup batteries as well.

Heart-related issues

Children who are born with or develop heart conditions that make it hard to breathe when they are physically active face challenges in engaging in vigorous outdoor activities. In the past, children with heart conditions often had many activity restrictions imposed on them, but now there is greater recognition that children with congenital heart disease also benefit from having active lifestyles that prevent long-term health complications. Your child with congenital heart disease would benefit from being outside every day. Their cardiologist should let you know if you need to restrict their activities and what signs to look for to make sure they are OK. We have both had patients with complex congenital heart disease, ones living extremely active lifestyles, athletes even, who have defied the odds of when they would need corrective surgery. The pediatric cardiologists and surgeons are especially proud of these active children and their families. Sometimes for children and families who have gone through significant medical histories, finding an outdoor activity to boost their spirits can be very helpful. Remember that even low-intensity activities in nature can provide many benefits.

Physical stamina

After a long period of inactivity, children who try to be active outside might describe shortness of breath. Maybe these children were sick or injured and unable to be active. Some children with rheumatologic, autoimmune, chronic pain, chronic fatigue, or endocrine disorders may have difficulty finding energy to participate in outdoor activities. Some children with chronic medical conditions may have trouble with temperature regulation and not have the stamina to participate in the way they choose. Or maybe a child became inactive, choosing playing computer games or reading books over being outside. For whatever reason, it can be hard for deconditioned children to become active outside, because it is, at first, so uncomfortable. At this point, your child may be self-restricting, feeling reluctant to participate. You will need to come up with a gradual plan to build up their strength, endurance, and confidence so they, too, can experience the joys that nature brings. This change is always easier for children if you can do the activity with them or bring along a supportive friend.

REFLECTION: If you have or care for a child who is not active outside because they are reluctant to go or because you worry about their medical condition, take a moment to explore these feelings. There are some very common conditions and less common ones where parents and caregivers may be particularly worried about their child engaging in outdoor, nature-based activities. Even if you wish for your child to participate, you may worry that being outdoors, especially being active outdoors, could be harmful. Discuss your concerns with your child's health care practitioner so they can advise whether a true activity restriction is needed or your child can fully participate in all activities but may just need their medications or other treatment plans adjusted. If there are restrictions on physical activity, you can still find less-active ways for your child to soak in nature (views, sounds, and smells) so they will remain safe.

The place to start is a series of conversations about a change in lifestyle. Be frank and open with even your youngest children.

- You want them to be as healthy and happy as possible, and being outside, including playing in nature, is an important part of that.
- Discuss what part of nature they may want to first explore, and talk about easy ways to access this.
- Let them choose the activity or give them a couple of options if they are uncertain. Start with one brief attempt, and talk about what went well and what did not go well.
- Set up a routine, then, of getting out once per week, adding more excursions as you can. Even if your child is old enough to not require supervision in this nature play, for reluctant, deconditioned children, you will probably have to do the nature play with them, encouraging them along the way.
- Another idea is to invite a close friend along to encourage their active play or sign up for an outdoor-oriented club or camp with them. And be sure to give your child lots of positive reinforcement for moving out of their comfort zone and challenging themselves.

Nature for Children With Sensory Disabilities

Children with visual or hearing disabilities may encounter additional safety concerns and challenges in navigating outdoor spaces. If your child uses hearing aids, it's important to make sure these devices are in good working condition and there are extra batteries available for any longer excursion. Extreme heat, cold, and precipitation can affect their functioning. For children who use glasses or contact lenses, similar guidance applies to make sure they have backup supplies for camping or other longer trips away from home. Children with blindness, deafness, or severe sensory disabilities can certainly experience nature with their other senses. Remember to look for local community groups and nonprofit groups that help children with physical disabilities experience nature. These groups usually have outdoor and nature programs for children with sensory disabilities as well. Parents and caregivers can focus on the rest of their child's senses to bring them nature experiences. Remember other senses, like smell and touch, when you are outside to enhance experiences for all ages and all abilities. Communicate with child care providers and school teachers about how your child can get more from their time outside.

Nature Nugget: Youth Employment Solutions Outdoors for the Blind

Every state has a federally funded vocational rehabilitation program to help people with disabilities (like vision loss or hearing loss) learn new skills and work on a vocational path. Check online for what is available in your state, or ask your local librarian to help you search.

Child who has blindness goes on a walk with her family.

Source: Jacobus tenBroek Library, National Federation of the Blind.

The Washington State Department of Services for the Blind (DSB) has a program for teens with low vision and blindness called Youth Employment Solutions. These are multi-week summer camps that focus on career exploration and preparation. DSB partners with employers and community groups to offer these experiences. One of the most popular and successful has been placing students who have low vision or who are blind with an all-outdoor preschool at the University of Washington Arboretum. To learn more, see the program brochure (https:// dsb.wa.gov/sites/default/files/public/services/documents/ YESBrochureWeb.pdf).

Nature for Children Who Have Significant Restrictions

Sometimes heart conditions cause dangerous problems when children are active. This category might include severe congenital deformities of the heart, when the child is waiting for or recovering from surgical repair, or electrical conditions of the heart, where physical activity can trigger the heart to beat erratically or even stop. Children who have had a recent concussion also need to limit strenuous activity and increase activity progressively with guidance from their medical team. This category might also include children whose body may be too frail to expend the energy needed for being physically active, like those with restrictive eating disorders or anorexia. Children with eating disorders may have to follow restrictions on how much physical activity they

Unearthing a New Hobby

A 12-year-old avid baseball player in my practice was diagnosed with a familial electrical problem in his heart. Both his mother's and sister's heart had previously stopped beating during exercise, but fortunately, it had been resuscitated. The young boy's cardiologist felt certain that he should *not* participate in baseball, or any usual, physically active sport, to prevent his heart from stopping. Fortunately, though, his cardiologist suggested fishing as a new "sport." The entire family was safe to participate, and this nature experience and sport became some of their favorite family time.

—Danette

can have so they do not expend too many calories. Being in nature, though, can be very helpful for their often coexisting depression or anxiety. We want parents of children who do have to have their physical activities restricted to get detailed instruction from their child's health care team. Find out if sitting outside to bird-watch or picnic is OK. Or, if not, you can set them up in a chair with an interesting nature view from a window or porch. These restrictions can be the beginning of a new hobby such as bird spotting or nature art. Once the child is cleared to increase their movement, nature walks or light gardening activities could be beneficial. Most of these children, with time, can eventually increase their activities outdoors, so always stay in communication with your child's health care team to know what is safe.

For eating disorders, nature time is sometimes seen as part of the treatment plan. An interesting strategy being used by some treatment programs and therapists is horticulture therapy. Horticulture therapy has been defined as the use of plants and plant-based activity for the purpose of human healing and rehabilitation. Depending on their stage in treatment, some patients may be able to engage in planting or harvesting a garden and then cooking. One program, available in a handful of states, known as the Walden program, refers to this as a "seed to table" approach. The National Eating Disorders Association encourages those with eating disorders to cook as a way to assist in their pathway to recovery and as a form of self-care, which is often low in those who struggle with an eating disorder. Cooking encourages us to slow down and focus on what we are eating and allows us to be more attuned to our hunger and fullness cues. As a result, we can engage in intuitive eating, which is something that individuals with eating disorders often have difficulty incorporating into their meals. You can find more information about horticulture therapy in eating disorder treatment by accessing the Walden program website (www.waldeneatingdisorders.com).

Nature for Children With Behavioral or Neurodevelopmental Conditions

Neurodivergent conditions and attention issues are very common. Each child's support needs are unique and affect their behavior. The level of these needs occurs on a spectrum from low to high, and even in the same child, many factors will lend themselves to "easy days" and "hard days." You know your child best and will need to advocate for the environmental and circumstantial qualities that are most likely to produce easier days in nature.

Attention-deficit/hyperactivity disorder

Parents and educators have often shared stories with us that children who have difficulty sitting still and being attentive indoors can often be well-behaved and focused when outdoors in nature. Research even shows that children with attention-deficit/hyperactivity disorder (ADHD) can concentrate better after spending time in nature. Yet if you are the parent of a child with ADHD, you might have extra concerns about your child's behavior and safety in certain outdoor settings. Some parents find it helpful to set ground rules before heading outdoors, building in extra time for transitions. For example, make a list of things your child needs to do to prepare for the outdoors or when it's time to pack up. You could use a watch or your phone's timer to let your child know when it's time to get ready to leave a playground or beach. Remember to praise your child when they behave well, including being kind to others, in order to reinforce those behaviors. If your child has difficulty participating in an organized school or community program because of their behavior, you could try to work with the organizers to see how you and the school can support your child better. Consider discussing with your child's health care practitioner if there are other strategies or medications that could be helpful so your child is able to get opportunities to

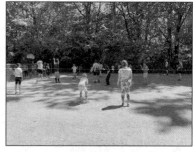

Outdoor game at Seattle's Apex Summer Camp.

ADHD Management

One of my 9-year-old patients had attention-deficit/hyperactivity disorder (ADHD) symptoms that often interfered with learning at school and making friends and contributed to impulsive behavior that landed him in trouble. Typical ADHD medications were tried, and although they did help with his attention and behavior, he had significant side effects. He experienced difficulty eating, weight loss, and slow growth. His parents eventually chose to stop the medications, take him out of school, and homeschool him. In addition to other behavioral supports, his mother told me that after much trial and error, they found he did very well if they worked on schoolwork for 15- to 30-minute increments, followed by time outside until he was ready to go back to work. Sometimes they were outside for only 10 minutes, but sometimes he would get very involved in something in their yard for over an hour. While many families may not have the opportunity or means to homeschool their child, make it a priority to explore whether an individualized education plan could include provisions for your child to take brief outdoor breaks that help them return and focus.

—Danette

be outdoors and in nature. Be sure to also work with your child's teacher to discover ways that nature exploration and outdoor time may enhance their instruction for your child. Finally, know that regular, one-on-one, child-directed special time is a widely recommended positive parenting strategy included in behavioral management programs for parents of children with ADHD. Try setting aside at least 15 minutes a week for some special outdoor time where your child decides what you both will do, and you give them your full, undistracted attention.

A wonderful example of a special program geared toward children with ADHD and autism spectrum disorder is the Apex Summer Camp in Seattle, WA. This is an evidence-based summer camp program focused on building social skills, positive relationships, and self-esteem within the context of structured recreational and learning activities. Children participate in typical camp activities, including outdoor sports and nature time, but all with small staff to camper ratios and supervision by trained staff aiming to make this a successful and positive experience for children. Check the offered programs in your area that have staff specially trained to work with children who have neurodivergent conditions.

Autism spectrum disorder

A child with autism may love the outdoors or they may be reluctant to engage with the different sensory experiences in an outdoor environment. As you plan time outside for your child with autism spectrum disorder, consider whether they will need extra supervision in case of wandering or if there is water nearby. In some cases, enjoying the outdoors is a learned behavior, so it is important to

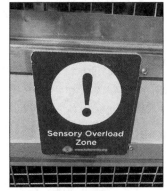

Sensory overload sign.

Lifestyle Strategies to Help With ADHD

In the past, I met 8-year-old twin boy patients who were struggling in school. Both had recently been diagnosed with attention-deficit/ hyperactivity disorder (ADHD), but one was having a harder time than the other. The frequent school meetings, doctors' appointments, and exhausting nightly behavioral challenges at home were taking a toll on the parents. In addition to their medications, it was suggested to them that they try enrolling the boys in a sports program, and the boys chose soccer. Within weeks, the parents noticed that their boys were completely different on the field and with their teams! Their mom described to me that their behavior not only improved on the field but was seemingly translating to being a little more settled at home and at school.

Although sports participation does not necessarily equate with time in nature, outdoor sports certainly give children the opportunity to move and play in ways that are not possible indoors. Plus, many fields are surrounded by trees and plants, with lots of sunshine and fresh air. For some children, having a more structured approach to play—and one that gives a bit of a break to their parents—may be a great solution for everyone in the family.

—Pooja

introduce your child to outside play for all the health and developmental benefits. If your child is reluctant to go outdoors, start by trying to relocate some favorite indoor activities to nearby outdoor spaces. Slowly, have them venture out farther. Water, sand, sidewalk chalk, and bubbles are all small ways to expose them to new sensory experiences. Many aquariums and museums provide nature exploration indoors. These places often have hours that are dedicated to people with sensory sensitivities, when they lower the lights or quiet the noises. They may also have signed locations that are away

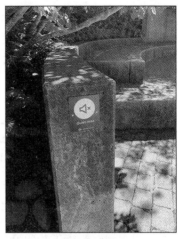

Quiet zone sign in a park.

from crowds for a child with this condition to spend a moment to regroup after sensory or emotional overload.

These strategies work and can be used in a park by going at hours when there are fewer people and looking for the quiet corners for a calming moment. Check in with your child's health care practitioner or therapist about other suggestions for how to safely have your child engage in nature-based experiences that are specific to your child and their needs.

Intellectual disabilities

There is a wide spectrum of abilities among children who have some type of intellectual disability that limits their cognitive functioning or ability to carry out some activities of daily life. Depending on their abilities, these children may face additional challenges participating in mainstream outdoor activities safely. This means that they are at higher risk of not meeting physical activity guidelines or engaging in health-promoting behaviors. It also means that safety must be considered. Parents and programs should provide supervision to meet their child's developmental level and their child's ability to judge the safety of settings and situations. Supporting these children to engage in nature-based activities and outdoor recreation, either individually or with a group program tailored for special needs, could have a profound impact on their health and well-being. Take a moment to plan for the level of supervision or environmental modifications that need to occur to make nature time safe for your child with an intellectual disability.

Nature for Children With Mental Health Issues

There is growing recognition of the benefits from nature contact for mental health. Time in nature reduces symptoms of anxiety and depression and can help children recover from trauma or illness. For a young person with depression, spending time in nature may reduce symptoms simply by getting them to move their body or may lift their mood because of the beauty and awe of the surroundings. Any type of nature experience can provide these types of benefits for those struggling with mental health issues.

The difficult part for families trying to immerse their child into nature when the child has mental health conditions is navigating their child's apathy or fear. Your child may not initially feel like they have the energy or desire to be outdoors because of their depressive symptoms. For a child with anxiety, you might encounter some resistance to going into nature if something about spending time outdoors increases their level of worry. If this is your situation, try encouraging them to start in locations that feel safe and comfortable to them, and spend brief amounts of time there until they feel ready to venture farther out and for longer. Combining other activities with outdoor time can also ease someone into nature time: having picnics, building snowmen,

Nature Nugget: Nature's Effect on Mood

Dr Greg Bratman at the University of Washington conducted studies that showed that the relationship between nature exposure and improved mental health may be at least partially a result of nature's impact on rumination, which is repetitive thinking or dwelling on negative feelings and distress and their causes and consequences. Heightened rumination has been shown to be associated with a negative mood and a greater risk of experiencing depression and anxiety. In a 2021 study with more than 600 adults, his team found that more average weekly time in nature was related to positive affect (state of mind) and less rumination. The next time you're in nature, try to be aware of your mood and thoughts and see if this could be a routine way to lift your spirits. Share this information with your child in an age-appropriate way to teach them strategies that can help them develop positive coping skills.

Source: Bratman GN, Young G, Mehta A, Babineaux IL, Daily GC, Gross JJ. Affective benefits of nature contact: the role of rumination. *Front Psychol.* 2021;12:643866.

drawing or coloring, taking photographs, and playing games on apps are all simple ways to combine these elements. Some mental health therapists are now incorporating horticulture or other nature-based strategies into their therapy with patients. We have seen many of our patients benefit from their time in nature. Evidence supports the idea that these children will feel better and appreciate the value of nature in their recovery and will perhaps build it into their repertoire of how to be resilient in the future. If your child is seeing a therapist for mental health conditions or symptoms, ask them for specific nature-time suggestions. There are also online resources dedicated to nature for children with mental health conditions.

Nature for Children Who Are Medically Fragile

The term *medically fragile* typically refers to children whose medical condition makes them more likely to have an adverse health event in typical surroundings. While we usually use this term for children with truly precarious medical conditions, it is also helpful to think about all medical conditions that may make parents fearful enough to keep their children from being outside. Some parts of nature exposure can be a problem for medically fragile children. Children with these conditions need nature time for their overall health and well-being just as much as any child, but with some careful preplanning.

This category includes children with the following conditions (but is not limited to these conditions):

- Cancer or immune system disorders that make them more vulnerable to infections
- Seizure disorders or epilepsy with a risk of getting seizures when they are overheated or dehydrated
- Lack of pigment in the skin to protect against injury from the sun
- Diabetes
- Food allergies and restrictions
- Conditions that predispose children to serious complications

Weakened immune system

Children with weaker immune systems are at higher risk of developing infections. These infections are often more dangerous to immunocompromised children than others. This adds a new level of worry and the need for protection from parents and caregivers. It is important to note, though, that viral and bacterial infections are more likely to be transmitted indoors and in places with more chances for transmission from other people. We remember

Navigating a New Diagnosis

I recently met the parent of a 6-year-old child with newly diagnosed type 1 diabetes. They had always enjoyed the outdoors as a family, but with this new diagnosis, they were nervous about venturing too far away from medical care. With the diagnosis, there were so many new things they had to think about (eg, checking blood sugar levels, managing insulin, watching for concerning symptoms) that they worried about taking hikes where they wouldn't have cell phone reception. Before the diagnosis, they used to camp a few times every summer, but now, they weren't sure how safe it would be to bring all the diabetes gear to a remote campground and worried about a possible emergency.

Fortunately, they sought out an endocrinologist who enjoyed the outdoors and appreciated what it meant for this family. He was able to provide both guidance and reassurance on how this new diagnosis, while it required special considerations, was not going to stop them from enjoying outdoor activities that they loved.

—Pooja

how liberating it was to learn that all of us were safer from COVID-19 when outside. We even started doing some patient visits in the parking lot!

Most children being treated for cancer have a weakened immune system from the medications they must take; some children with autoimmune conditions are also taking medications that make it difficult to fight infections, and some children are born with a weak immune system. Nature provides all the benefits to these children and families too, including helping with the stress of managing these complicated conditions. While care must be taken to reduce the risk for infections from others, outdoor time is generally the safest way to be with others. We know about the fear of infection that families carry, but try to expand the experiences of a child with an immunocompromising condition. Playdates outside may be the only socializing considered safe. Even when your child is hospitalized, look for nature. Some children's hospitals have patios and gardens that patients can use. Look for seats with an outdoor view during infusions. Be sure to ask your child's health care team for these things if you don't find them. While you can discuss with your child's health care team what types of outdoor activities can be safely pursued by your

A Blooming Social Life While Battling Cancer

I had a 6-year-old patient battling an aggressive form of leukemia. He and his family were diligent with his treatment. It was very hard on the family and his 9-year-old brother. His mother often appeared exhausted and shared her concerns about the whole family with me. At one visit, she came in excited to share that they were all doing better.

A big part of the problem was the restrictions placed on her boys of not being able to spend time with their friends because the younger brother's immune system was weakened from chemotherapy and bone marrow transplant. After they had discussed this with the cancer treatment team, they were given the green light to socialize outside. The family began eating dinner outside every day they could, and once or twice per week, they had playdates with the boys' friends and family, in all weather. The boy's mother really noticed a difference in everyone's attitude once they were able to make nature a priority.

—Danette

child, know that most of the time, the outdoors will be safer than indoors for infection risk.

Seizures and epilepsy

We have known families that limited their children from playing outdoors for fear of increased seizures or did not let their child with a seizure disorder near water and swimming because they feared it may be too big of a risk. These children should not be around water, swim, or do any water sports alone. But most of these risks can be mitigated with careful planning and supervision. Having a seizure during time within the water or near it can be dangerous, so these children should have adult attention on them, with an adult close enough to intervene immediately if needed. For children with frequent seizures, this is likely to mean someone in addition to a lifeguard, who divides their attention across all swimmers in the water. Life jackets, appropriately sized and fastened correctly, are essential.

Although not true for all children with seizures or epilepsy, heat and dehydration can trigger an episode. Heat and dehydration can also trigger a crisis for children with sickle cell anemia and other blood conditions. Nature time

---

Heat-Triggered Seizures

For a patient of mine with a significant seizure disorder and other health conditions, overheating often triggered seizures. Her school eventually stopped sending her out for recess, but this precaution made her upset and withdrawn. She wanted to be outside with her friends. Her parents worked hard to figure out what outdoor temperature seemed to trigger her seizures. Then, every 3 years when I would rewrite her individualized education plan for school, her parents and I included the importance of letting her go outside every day as long as the heat index was less than 80°. Like many other conditions, your child's specific condition doesn't have to prevent them from enjoying nature entirely. With the right tools and precautions, there are many ways they can still enjoy nature while staying safe.

—Danette

---

for these children should always include a plan for repeated water breaks and keeping an eye on the outdoor temperature. Cooling vests and scarves may be helpful. These strict plans should be shared with the school, child care, and youth programs that these children attend. With careful planning and communication with others in your child's life, your child, too, can enjoy nature time.

Vitiligo and albinism

Conditions that leave the skin completely unprotected from the sun because there is no pigment also require special considerations for time outdoors.

Sometimes this lack of pigment affects a child's entire body (albinism) and sometimes it occurs just in small spots (vitiligo). Either way, areas without any pigment can more easily develop skin cancer from sun exposure. And because the danger is from repeated exposure, even on cloudy days, parents and caregivers are sometimes fearful of outdoor time for these children. Access to time outside begins with the strategies all of us must abide by when exposed to the sun's harmful rays:

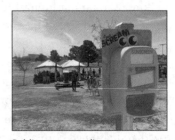

Public sunscreen dispenser.

Source: Photo by Brenda Maxon and available at www.cdc.gov/skin-cancer/stories.

reduce midday exposure and time in direct sunlight and use high-protection sunscreen applied correctly. What children in our care with albinism also do when outside is wear SPF-rated clothes and hats as well as sunglasses with UV protection. These clothes and glasses are easily available. It can be difficult to see with dark sunglasses on cloudy days, but using photochromic or transition lenses that darken as the day brightens helps this work more efficiently. I (DG) cared for a nature-loving family with a daughter who had albinism that moved to Seattle to feel more comfortable being outside in the lower-risk cloudy days. We are not recommending that families with these conditions move to manage the sun but recommending that children continue to play in the shade when possible and never miss going out in the rain and on cloudy days. With all the protections in place, there is no reason to limit outdoor time. Again, always ensure that child care and school follow your preferred protection plan.

Conditions that predispose to serious complications

Risks related to minor injuries or falls take on extra significance when your child has a condition that puts them at high risk of bleeding easily or fracturing their bones. The parts of nature play that make it good for development, such as the uneven terrain and risky play, can frighten families into keeping children with these conditions indoors. The good thing is that nature-based activities can be tailored to mitigate risks. We suggest slowly introducing your child to trying safer activities with supervision, and protective gear could help them become more adept at participating in those activities. Noncontact and low-impact activities like hiking, fishing, golf, and swimming pose low risk for children with conditions that predispose them to serious injuries. Also, look for playgrounds with spongy, springy ground cover around play equipment. Children can lose their coordination and good judgment when they become tired, so it is wise to watch for this as well.

Diabetes

Some children with diabetes (and their parents), especially those who require close monitoring of their glucose levels and insulin, may feel reluctant to go on outdoor excursions that take them away from medical services. Many of the linked glucose monitors and insulin pumps also require internet access to correctly monitor and dose insulin, so families and older children need to understand backup plans to use finger sticks and a plan for dosing. Plus, glucose and insulin levels can differ when children are exerting themselves

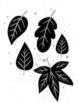

Summer Camp for Children With Special Health Care Needs

Many children's hospitals or other condition-specific organizations sponsor sleepover summer camps for children with special health care needs, such as for diabetes, heart conditions, autism spectrum disorder, sickle cell disease, neurological disorders, genetic conditions, and others. They are usually staffed by many physicians, nurses, and other health care professionals. For children who have health care conditions that require diligent monitoring and adjusting, such as diabetes or heart conditions, summer camp is usually out of the question. But special camps such as these offer children with these serious conditions a chance to be around their peers in nature while also receiving the specialized care they need.

When volunteering one year, I had a 9-year-old camper with diabetes share with me that her camp time was "the best-ever time in the whole world!" I have no doubt that this experience will long be remembered by her.

—Pooja

in outdoor activities or spending time in the outdoor heat or cold. These are valid concerns, and each child's body is different in how it responds. Yet it is even more important for long-term cardiovascular health that children with diabetes be regularly physically active. We suggest considering the monitoring of blood sugar levels and dosing of insulin whenever your child starts a new activity. This is especially important for outdoor activities, when a low or high environmental temperature can complicate management, such as a new sport, a summer camp, or a family camping trip. You should make a checklist to help remember to pack all medications and monitoring devices for your outdoor excursions and include supplies for backup plans. As your child gets older, you'll want to help them become more aware of signals from their body and learn how to respond if they don't feel well. They will gradually learn to take over this planning for an active life.

Food restrictions

One of the most common chronic health conditions that occur in children is food allergies and other medical conditions that are managed with food restrictions. While we don't expect food restrictions to affect a child's outdoor

Feasting Outdoors

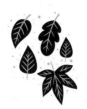

For some families, food is a core part of outdoor excursions—and I come from one of them! When I was growing up, visits to local, state, and national parks always included special food and drinks. This meant we usually had things like a pot of rice and vegetables, potato-stuffed parathas (Indian bread), and a large thermos of hot chai with us. Before or after a hike, family and friends would set up a potluck at a picnic table and enjoy the outdoor setting. Even now, we can count on my mom to bring along little pouches of nuts or other treats with her that keep the grandchildren happy during our outdoor family meetups.

In my 20s, I went on my first camping trip to an island in the middle of Lake George, NY, with a large group of friends. The campsite was very rustic, but the meal was elaborate—chickpea curry, tandoori chicken, and naan! I was given the role of chopping vegetables, while the more experienced outdoor chefs tackled the cooking. This is why hot dogs and prepackaged meals don't quite cut it for me when on an outdoor adventure! Even if I am packing sandwiches for a hike, I like to think of what else will feel special when we finally sit down to rest and eat—perhaps some chilled grapes, spicy chips, or sparkling water to elevate the meal.

My memories may resonate with some of you, while others may prefer to keep things as simple as possible during nature excursions. I wanted to share this with you in case some members of your family or friend group are different from you in how they think about food for outdoor events. A reluctant child may be more likely to enjoy their nature experience if you plan, pack, and eat some of their favorite foods. Others may feel overwhelmed by extensive food planning and want to keep things easy. One thing is likely universal, though: having a full belly and staying hydrated will make any experience go more smoothly for people of all ages!

—Pooja

activities, we know of many examples where parents have restricted or considered restricting activities because of their concerns related to their child being able to eat safely.

If your child has food allergies, food protein–induced enterocolitis syndrome, celiac disease, or other dietary restrictions, you are used to worrying about them being able to have food that is safe and appropriate for them. You might wonder whether you should let them go on a school overnight trip, to a summer camp, or on a camping weekend with friends. We have patients whose parents have had their children miss out on these memorable opportunities because they didn't feel safe about the food environment. We want to empower you to advocate for your child having their dietary needs met so they are not excluded from these outdoor opportunities. Most schools, child

---

Gluten-Free Adventures

My son has celiac disease, which means he cannot eat any gluten-containing foods, such as wheat, barley, or rye. In middle school, he had a school trip scheduled to Oregon that involved many outdoor experiences, such as hiking, white water rafting, and snowshoeing. This would be the first time he was away from us for that long since being diagnosed with celiac disease. We had become used to reading labels, researching restaurants in advance, and asking a lot of questions about menu items to make sure he could eat safely when outside the home. But now we were worried that he or his trip chaperones would not be able to do all this during the school trip. His gastroenterologist had encouraged us to help our son learn and practice being the person reading labels and asking questions at restaurants, so he could become more confident doing so.

We also set up a meeting with the school contact person in charge of logistics and meals and were pleased with their thoughtful approach. The school had already planned where the students would be eating each meal and were able to request or pull up online the menus from each place to identify that gluten-free options were available. In one case where there wasn't a good option, they helped identify another nearby restaurant where one chaperone would go to pick up a meal for my son. Finally, they allowed us to send some additional snacks that he could have with him in his backpack in case there were unexpected challenges in getting gluten-free food. These additional steps took time and resources but helped make for a successful and memorable school trip for my son.

—Pooja

care, or community programs should be able to reassure you that they will have food that is specifically allergen-free or meets restrictions for diets such as vegetarian, halal, or kosher. At other times, you might need to educate them about what foods are permissible for your child to eat and maybe even help do some research about food options that are available where they are going or send food along that you know your child can eat. For older children, help them practice advocating for themselves in situations when you are not around to be able to identify and ask for foods that they are allowed to eat. If your child has been prescribed medications including an EpiPen and antihistamine for their food allergies, please make sure you send all of those along, including a detailed care plan for if there is an exposure. Check the Food Allergy Research and Education website (www.foodallergy.org) for parent support and tools for managing any specific food-restricting condition.

Inclusive Nature and Outdoors

According to the Centers for Disease Control and Prevention, since nearly 27% of children have a chronic health condition, it is important to consider how to make nature experiences inclusive, safe, and enjoyable for these children. With some extra planning and consideration of special health care needs, all children can and should experience meaningful time in nature. It may take some additional effort to find outdoor spaces that are accessible and advanced planning to make sure you have what you need to feel safe and comfortable. There are many partners that can make this happen, so gather a list of local community groups, parks programs, and other resources. All children benefit from time outdoors, especially in nature, and we are hopeful that with the tips and activities suggested in this chapter, each of you can find a way to make that happen safely and comfortably for your family.

Nature and the Early Years: Birth Through Age 5

Nature and the Early Years: Birth Through Age 5

When you take your child for a well-child checkup, one of the most important evaluations focuses on how they are advancing in their developmental milestones. You might be worried about whether your child is progressing at the right pace, how they compare to other children, and what you could be doing differently to support their development. We both remember nervously waiting for our pediatrician to announce what they thought about our children's progress, even though we are both primary care pediatricians ourselves!

Healthy children follow a fairly predictable developmental trajectory. This includes the development of gross motor or big muscle skills with increasing strength and then the perfection of coordination. It also includes the development of fine motor skills, or using fingers with increasing precision, and then the perfection of this with writing and drawing. It includes the development of speech and then understanding and, eventually, the ability to read and communicate complex ideas. There is the advancement of cognitive abilities that allow the child to learn math and be able to plan, reason, and make good judgments. And there is the social-emotional development that progresses best in safe, stable, nurturing environments and lays the foundation for good mental health. The Centers for Disease Control and Prevention has easy-to-use developmental trackers, including checklists and an app, for children up to age 5 years.

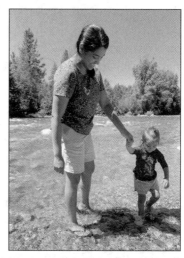
Taking a stroll along the river.

Young children gain developmental milestones but not on their own. Their environment and their relationships play major roles, and this is where time in nature can be critical for promoting many aspects of your child's development. Even if your child is on an atypical developmental trajectory, time in nature can be an excellent way to provide opportunities to enhance their development. This chapter outlines how to help promote and nurture developmental skills for infants, toddlers, and preschoolers through nature connection and time outdoors. Although it's not an exhaustive list, we've compiled some ideas that we recommend in our practices as well as some that we, personally, found to be successful as we raised our own children.

Infants and Toddlers

The effect nature has is magical and important for all children, but for the youngest, like infants and toddlers, it is especially powerful and long-lasting. Early brain science shows that the human brain is continually growing and making neuronal connections, called *synapses,* faster for 0- to 3-year-olds than for children of any other age. And by age 3 years, each of us has had the most connections we will ever have. After age 3 years, there is pruning of the connections that don't get used. Thus, your young child needs time in nature to influence this brain development. These natural world experiences have more effect on the young, developing brain and set the stage for lifelong health and learning. Early family habits are lasting habits, although it is never too late to start regular nature play. You can find out more about your child's early brain development from the Harvard University Center on the Developing Child (https://developingchild.harvard.edu).

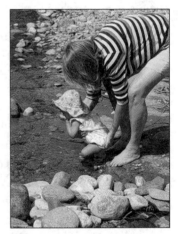

Danette and her granddaughter taking a dip in the river.

Make your outings in nature part of your family's routine. Starting from a young age, routines are great for children—something they can count on. When you take your baby outside for nature time, it can be helpful to have them in a front pack, backpack, or stroller. Even if your toddler is reliably walking, they can tire quickly, so consider having a stroller or wagon for them. Each time you step outdoors with your small child is an opportunity to connect with nature, even if it's as simple as noticing the sky.

Babies and toddlers are constantly changing, gaining new skills and growing. Sometimes it might feel like this growth happens overnight! Encouraging them to practice and have new experiences can help development stay on track. Don't be surprised by your toddler trying out their new skills in nature, over and over (such as moving 2 or 3 small rocks a short distance, back and forth, back and forth). I (DG) remember wondering if there was something different with my own children at this stage for "practicing" developmental skills over and over. Playing in nature and providing new experiences also encourage their emerging imagination. My (DG) son's 3-year-old friend announced that a fallen, hollow log was now his "fort" even though he could not get into or onto it! He simply wanted to be around it and imagine it as a fort. Toddlers love imaginary play!

Practice Makes Perfect

A friend of mine sent me a video of her 17-month-old grandson, John. This delightful video shows John in a raincoat and boots, walking into a small pile of wet leaves. You hear him ooh and ahh as he very gingerly tries out walking onto the leaves. At the end of the pile, he quickly turns around and steps back onto the pile, this time a little less carefully. Again, at the end he whips around to go back over the leaves. He moves back and forth, back and forth, getting faster and more confident and laughing and enjoying the fun until he marches right over the pile! John was persistent, practicing his big muscle skill set, over and over, until he was good at it—and all with a pile of leaves as the inspiration.

—Danette

Infant and toddler language development

The first 3 years after your child's birth are the most intensive and important period for developing speech and language skills. It is no surprise that babies develop best when they are surrounded by an environment full of sights, sounds, and interactions with others. During these years, most infants will progress from using gestures and body language, to babbling and cooing, to saying their first words, to being able to put words together into sentences. Interacting with nature can promote your young child's language development. As soon as you are outside, notice the sights, sounds, smells, and feel of the weather—rain, sun, breeze, and cool or warm air. Describe all of these to your young child and ask them questions.

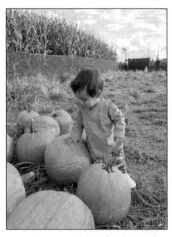

"I see that the big tree across the street is dropping leaves. Let's see what colors the leaves are!"

"Smell how fresh the air is after the rain? Take a deep breath!"

Don't forget to point out the sky with interesting clouds, the sun and moon, birds and planes, and more.

Which is your favorite pumpkin?

"I hear those loud birds again… Caw! Caw! I see 1-2-3 birds! Can you make the sound of a bird?"

New experiences in nature encourage communication between you and your child. Hearing your voice as you narrate nature time is a delight for babies and toddlers. You also model curiosity about and respect for the natural world when you do this. Sing simple songs about the outdoors, and encourage older infants and toddlers to sing along. Watch your child's facial expressions to know when they especially enjoy what you are doing or when they are not enjoying the experience. These interactions teach them ways to experience nature as well as promote language and communication.

We know that young children who are exposed to more than one language are better learners later in school. Studies have shown that dual language learners can have better executive function that supports their focus, memory, and decision-making. Also, these children learn other languages more quickly. Be sure to use all languages you use at home in your nature interactions from a young age, and encourage other caregivers to do this as well. Even if you have some familiarity with another language, look up some nature words (eg, *animals, trees, moon, sun*) and use them with your child. I (PT) spoke to my children exclusively in Hindi when they were toddlers and have an adorable video of my 2-year-old son telling me in Hindi about 2 duckies on a lake. I also remember going back and forth in Hindi about "What does a cat say? What does a doggie say?" and so on with a long list of animals. While our family eventually transitioned to a primarily English-speaking household as the kids became older, I really encourage those of you who can to keep the multiple languages as part of your daily communication for as long as possible.

Infant and toddler fine motor or small muscle development

Developmentally, this age-group likes to reach and touch objects. Children this age will even explore objects with their mouth. Make sure to offer safe, natural items to touch and explore. While you can set your baby down on various kinds of surfaces, be careful the surface is not hot, sharp, or something they can roll off of and hurt themselves. Have your infant and toddler touch and feel all kinds of textures that are smooth, rough, hard, soft, wet, and so on. Try offering them bits of grass, rocks, leaves and pine cones, and dirt to explore with their hands. If it's winter and you live in an area where snow accumulates, introduce them to snow angels or have them catch snowflakes with their tongue (tasting snow is OK as long as it is fresh and not dirty in any way). I (PT) loved seeing a video of a little one "playing in the snow" indoors with his grandmother, who creatively placed a small heap of snow onto a metal tray for an indoor winter activity. Whether you're inside or outside, start conversations with your child as they focus on what's in their hands. Describe what it is and see how they react. These can also lead to very cute pictures and videos! Reaching, pointing, and practicing a fine pincer grasp should be part of this exploring to encourage fine motor skills. Make sure you watch your child closely as they explore small items and ensure they don't put them into their mouth. When your child is done exploring, make sure they wash their hands with soap and water afterward before they eat or put their hands into their mouth. When they're old enough to eat pieces of fruits and vegetables, talk about how those foods grow on plants or trees and have your child touch the surfaces of whole fruits and vegetables. Older toddlers might even be able to help you pick some berries or tomatoes, if that's an activity available to you.

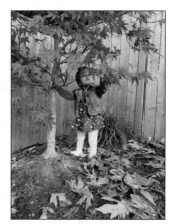

Enjoying the fall leaves.

Digging Into Nature

Toddlers can stay entertained for a long time if they have the opportunity to dig, such as in a sandbox or on a real beach, helping promote their fine and gross motor skills. In addition to a shovel, grab some other small containers (even washed-out plastic yogurt containers) or sand toys for them to have more opportunities to dig, fill, and build structures. If there is a pool or water nearby, you can teach them how to safely collect and transport that water for more fun, teaching them to also hone their balance skills as they try not to spill. If they play with their siblings or friends, they'll also get to practice their communication and social interactions. Bring a blanket or chair for yourself and enjoy these moments with your child as they enjoy playing and developing many skills. This was a favorite activity for my boys and a perfect way to spend a warm weekend afternoon.

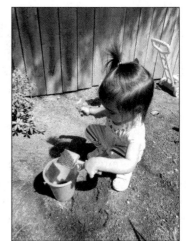

—Pooja

Infant and toddler gross motor or big muscle development

Encourage your infant to scoot and roll on different natural surfaces, such as sand, grass, or even snow. You could have them sit or roll on a picnic blanket after making sure there is nothing sharp underneath. Support your toddler as they try to stand, walk, run, or climb on and kick at these different textured surfaces. This activity supports and promotes their gross motor or big muscle skills. At first your child may hesitate, but then they will do more,

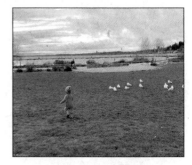

Running in a field with seagulls.

gaining confidence as they try again and again. In the city, you can have your toddler try stepping between sidewalks and grates, pavement and tree wells, and gravel and mud puddles. Exploring sensations outdoors is also fun if you have access to a swing, especially a small harness swing for toddlers and infants who can sit up. Many parks with play equip-

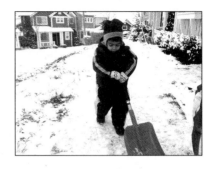

ment have these special swings. Start slow and work up to faster. Talk about the wind rushing by and the excitement of moving fast on a swing. Take cues from your child and slow down when they look scared or are not enjoying the activity. If you have access to only a regular swing, hop on yourself and hold your young child tight. Be careful, though, not to go down a slide holding your infant or toddler, as they can get injured if their arm or leg gets caught, so it's safer to enjoy slides only when they are old enough to go down alone. You could bring a ball to a park or other grassy area and they could learn to roll back and forth or throw and kick. If you have a garden or indoor plants, have your toddler help you water them with a small container of water that is easy for them to lift. Encourage them to use small tools such as a shovel or rake (or even an old spoon) to dig and explore the sand or dirt. All this moving, shoveling, and balancing with tools helps with their big muscle skills.

Infant and toddler cognitive development

Play is how children learn. This shockingly simple statement has been studied and validated in scientific research and is now the emphasis for many child development specialists. And, when the adults in a young child's life join them in play, these joyful interactions are even more powerful in building cognitive skills, along with language, social-emotional skills, and self-regulation. Sometimes we think that play is frivolous, but it actually enhances brain structure and promotes executive function, which is the basis for essential lifelong skills such as understanding priorities, setting goals, and managing time. Play has even been declared a fundamental right by the United Nations Convention on the Rights of the Child. Being outside and in nature makes playing easier, with all the interesting small bits, such as rocks and bugs, wind and weather, puddles, and mud. It sparks movement and imagination and certainly promotes joyful exploration, whether in the city or country, in all weather.

Going on a Dinosaur Hunt

When my son was a toddler, he became obsessed with dinosaurs. Those were all he wanted to talk about and all he wanted to pretend play. One day, when he was reluctant to go outside, I told him we were going to look for dinosaurs, and that got him going. We approached every bush and tree to look for dinosaurs. Of course, there weren't any and I noticed he became skeptical. Quickly, I got his interest again when I picked up pine cones and small rocks, declaring that we had found dinosaur eggs. He was thrilled, and every time we went outside during his dino phase, we repeated this ritual. He wanted to go outside more to find the "dinosaur eggs," and he started to make plans about where to look. His play now included planning and pretending, which promote cognitive skills.

—Danette

In nature, playfully encourage your child's cognitive development by creating games that promote brain development: hide a small rock under one of several leaves and ask your baby or toddler where it is. Encourage your toddler to find different colored flowers, or hide small toys for them to find in dirt, leaves, or snow or under bushes. Check first to make sure there are no thorns in the bushes. Consider bringing indoor toys outdoors to encourage outdoor play. Children will find it fun to play with their cars, trucks, dolls, kitchen sets, blocks, and other favorite toys in a new setting. Pretend play can become much more elaborate outdoors. Run and jump into a pile of leaves, into a snowbank, or into a rain puddle, asking your child to copy you. Have your older toddler rake or dig weeds and rocks. Count the trees or bushes on your block as you walk or run errands. Definitely show older infants and toddlers how to use tools, such as a garden spade, to dig and bury things. Show them how to use a magnifying glass to study plants, flowers, insects, rocks, ice, and more. Show them how to use sidewalk chalk if you have access to concrete or blacktop in a safe place. Be sure to ask them what they are drawing. Blow bubbles with bubble soap and describe how the wind carries them away or how they freeze. Encourage your toddler to choose small, easy-to-carry things for a collection, such as rocks, leaves, or flowers. Bring them home and keep them in a special place to look at later or use for art projects. Encourage your toddler to talk about their collections with others. Older toddlers love imaginative play, so pretend to be your child's favorite animal, prowling around outside. Hunt for dinosaurs or their other favorite imaginary characters. They may even enjoy dressing up as a favorite animal or character when they go for a walk or trip to the park. Tapping into our inner child and playing this way when our children were young (and now with grandchildren) is not only important for the child but also one of the best parts of parenting and grandparenting.

Infant and toddler social-emotional development

We cannot protect our children from all stressful situations, and we should not shield them from all stress, but we can make them resilient. They can be prepared to weather stressful times and situations much better. Your love, time, and attention help create these essential skills. Nature is the perfect

Nature Nugget: Growing Relationships

Have you heard of the term *early relational health*? Pediatricians like us are very excited about research showing that the relationship you forge with your infant and young child makes them healthier and happier throughout their life! This magic ingredient for children can happen with parents, grandparents and other relatives, and even child care providers and teachers.

Relationships, especially early in life, are biological necessities to build a foundation of lifelong growth and development. The best relationships are **safe** (free from physical or psychological harm; children believe their caregivers will protect them), **stable** (the adult is dependably there for the child), and **nurturing** (adults use warmth and clear expectations with their child).

Time outside in nature is the perfect setting to offer joy, awe, and wonder while you interact and grow your relationship with your young child. If not all relationships are ideal, time in nature could also be a way to build resilience and buffer the impact of challenging childhood circumstances. Check out the Harvard University Center on the Developing Child (https://developingchild.harvard.edu) and Zero To Three (www.zerotothree.org) for additional information for parents and caregivers.

setting for you and your child to build a safe, stable, and nurturing relationship. There is so much to do, see, and interact with in nature.

Young children are also learning to regulate their moods and emotions. Going outside is the perfect distraction that a cranky toddler needs to reduce tantrums. Parents and caregivers can also recharge their emotional well-being in nature. Taking care of an infant or a toddler is hard work, so you need nature time as well. When your little one is safely engaged outdoors or tucked into a stroller, you might have a few moments to feel the sunshine or fresh winter air, take a few breaths, and clear your mind. For grandparents or others helping care for your child, having them take a stroller walk with your baby or throw down a blanket to play on can be an easy way to get some outdoor time.

Head outside with your young child with the following activities in mind: Find a safe, interesting place to rest, then encourage your mobile infant or toddler to explore. You will notice that they often stick very close by at first. One way toddlers build their social-emotional resilience is by conquering their separation anxiety, a common fear that is often heightened at about 15 months of age. Pediatricians know that the 15- to 18-month well-child checkup may be very difficult, as a fearful toddler may cling to their parent and scream when they are examined. As with other developmental steps, toddlers work through this fear with practice in safe situations. When you are outside, they may slowly venture away, checking back in with you frequently. You will often see a child working on this dance of venturing out a few steps and then running back to safety at their parent's legs. If you see your child going too far, guide them back and start over. This is a great opportunity to teach them about feeling reassured, following instructions, and staying safe. Encourage them with words and touch as they explore and talk about their nature time later when you are back home. Talking about the day's activities is a perfect part of a bedtime routine, including discussing the emotions that the outdoor time brought up. You might recap a stressful moment with "We had so much fun at the park today, but when that dog came near, you were scared and ran back to me! But you were safe, and we could keep playing."

Nature and Child Care

For most young children who attend child care and preschool, it is important that there is outdoor and nature time each day. Studies confirm that when children are outside, they are more active, developing their muscles and

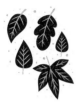

Playing in Puddles

When I was working on a research study to encourage physical activity and outdoor time in preschoolers, one of the child care centers was dealing with a difficult play-ground situation. The uneven ground led to the creation of a huge puddle during weeks of rainy weather. It was right next to the play structure and affecting the children's ability to run and use the whole space during their outdoor playtimes. The wonderful consultant we had working with the center for this study came up with the awesome idea of treating the puddle as they would a sensory water table!

After determining it was safe to do so, the center staff went ahead with this suggestion. They delightedly shared a video of the children dressed up in rainsuits and boots, engaged in playing in and around the puddle with little buckets. This was such a heartwarming example of turning lemons into lemonade…*or* puddles into play areas!

—Pooja

coordination. We also know that time in nature improves concentration and reduces behavioral problems. Child care and preschool teachers have known this even before studies confirmed it. Check with your child's program. Does the curriculum include nature topics? Are some of the children's books about nature topics? How often and how much are the children outside, including babies? Do they go outside in all kinds of weather, helping families provide weather-appropriate clothes like boots and rain jackets? Maybe they even provide outdoor gear for the students and teachers. Does the outdoor space include natural features that encourage nature play? This setup might include pathways looping through natural landscapes with native plants to support pollinators, boulders, dirt, and logs. Many child care programs plant vegetable gardens to supplement their food programs and involve the children in the process. Some educators will even bring nature elements indoors to support sensory experiences with things such as sand, leaves, and dried flowers.

Even if your child's program does not currently have a nature focus, ask the director what families can do to support them in creating these opportunities for children. Maybe offer to help organize a fundraising event to support the purchase of a nature curriculum or a nature workshop for early care and education providers. Some sites don't have covered areas that make it easier for children to go outdoors in all weather conditions, so parents could work to provide this setting. Many cities and states, in addition to the federal government and Head Start, are quite supportive of child care nature opportunities. Some areas have child care grants that provide money and programming to support outdoor and nature enhancements to child care. Look for local and state grants that are growing in availability throughout the country. Help your child's early care and education program apply for these funds. Don't forget to partner with local parks or other community programs that may bring opportunities to child care settings or can support nearby field trips. Rally and organize other parents to help develop a vegetable garden program or add natural elements to the indoor or outdoor play area. Some programs have been successful in collecting donations of plants, logs, and materials to create a raised garden bed.

The ultimate nature experiences in early childhood are nature, forest, or outdoor-focused groups or schools. These are grassroots programs that are set entirely or nearly all outside, in a natural setting, and have been popular in many places around the world, especially in Scandinavia and Germany (*Waldkindergarten* is the term used in Germany) and now in the United States.

The Fiddleheads Forest Preschool, located in Seattle's Washington Park Arboretum, even has children nap outside, calling it "cozy time." These schools are known to help children develop resilience, leadership, problem-solving, and perseverance. And these children are just as kindergarten ready as the children attending traditional, indoor centers. The state of Washington has developed licensing requirements for these child care settings to ensure a baseline of quality and safety, and many other states are following soon. These nature-immersion schools truly embrace the idea that there is no bad weather, and they seek to encourage unstructured, child-directed play in all types of climates. Most of these programs offer outdoor clothing and gear libraries so growing children are provided with all the rain, snow, and other extreme weather clothes they need to be comfortable and safe. Parents are given guidance about dressing their young children comfortably for the weather. The Natural Start Alliance, an organization uniting more than 1,000 nature-based and outdoor organizations, published in a report in 2022 that there are more than 800 outdoor preschools in the United States.

Preschoolers

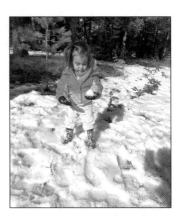

Preschool-aged children thrive in the outdoors. Their developmental skills make exploring and interacting with nature a little easier than for babies and toddlers. Plus, most preschoolers want to go outside. Your preschool-aged child may actually pester you to go out and then resist heading back inside. Most experts recommend at least 1 hour each day outdoors. Some days, you and your child's caregivers are just not going to be able to do this. One way to increase time in nature is to take your indoor activities outside. Nearly every part of your child's day can be enjoyed in nature rather than inside. This is easiest when the temperature outside is comfortable for the coats and hats you have. We encourage you to think about what indoor activities you can bring outdoors—playing, reading, socializing, learning, eating, and more! With more space to move and even get messy, you might find that both you and your preschooler are happier and calmer when outside. During precipitation, taking inside activities outside will be easiest if you have a covered area to protect you from rain or snow. Look for public spaces that have a covered area if you don't have this near home. Parks, schoolyards, or libraries are all ideas for finding a covered play area. Snowsuits and rain jackets and pants also help extend your options during rain and snow seasons.

You can do much more elaborate exploring in nature at this age because preschoolers have so many more skills. At this stage, a preschool-aged child needs less direct supervision than infants and toddlers. Your preschooler should understand about staying close, but they still need an adult nearby because they have not yet fully grasped what situations may be dangerous to them. Preschoolers may run after wildlife or jump from a too-high location

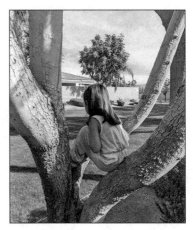

A fun outdoor adventure can include exploring trees.

or into water, trust strangers, or touch something sharp or hot. Despite this need for careful watching, this is your child's opportunity to take small risks and learn new skills and confidence. Encourage your preschooler to climb the playground ladder, jump into the pool or pile of snow, dig in the warm sand, and throw a ball. Use your judgment to make sure that these risks are not dangerous. The confidence and persistence your child learns from finally succeeding after 3 or 30 tries are priceless. Your support and encouragement during these attempts deepen your relationship as well.

Every day, preschool-aged children are developing new skills, including trying to be more independent. Nature time absolutely helps promote developmental milestones. But parents and other caregivers play a part, moving these young, curious children outside and helping them have fun in nature.

Child-directed versus adult-directed nature play

You can think about your preschooler's nature play in 2 ways: *child-directed* and *adult-directed*. Child-directed nature play is just that: the child decides what and where to explore with minimal parent/caregiver direction (but always with age-appropriate supervision). An example of this is sending your preschooler outside to play in your yard or going to a park and letting them loose. Both examples still require parent/caregiver supervision, and may even involve that you brainstorm what they can do when out in nature, but your child needs little direction from you about what they do once you are both outside. Adult-directed nature play is planned and executed by you. It could be scouring an outdoor space for bugs to put into a jar, side by side with your little one, or picking flowers and plants to study with a magnifying glass. Each activity includes you guiding the conversation about what your child sees and feels. Infants and toddlers need nearly all adult-guided nature play since you need to watch them so closely. Preschoolers benefit from both types of nature play. Remember to craft these opportunities with joy in mind. In either type of play, you can coax your little one to notice the awe of nature and engage with joy and emerging confidence.

Imaginary play

One of the best characteristics of preschool-aged children is their imagination! By the time a child is 3 years old, their neurons have made the most interconnections they will ever have, making them incredibly imaginative. This is the age of imaginary friends and the age of elaborately interactive play. Nature time feeds their imagination, and they can carry their imaginative

Finding Flower Fairies

One of my earliest memories is visiting the grand house and large-walled garden at my great aunt and uncle's farm when I was 4 years old. We lived in a very small house with a tiny yard at the time, so their farm and flower garden were fantastic to me. While the grown-ups sat around the kitchen talking, I was allowed to play outside as long as I stayed within the walls of the flower garden. The wall was about only 2–3 feet high, so of course I walked on the top around the whole perimeter, which was thrilling. Within the garden were flowering plants, and I searched hard for flower fairies. This was a magical place, made so much more special by my imaginative play, and has stayed with me years later.

—Danette

storylines to the outdoors. They may act out these storylines alone or may enjoy having you join them. Their memory and their understanding of the concept of the future help with this too. Read a book about dinosaurs or fairies, then make plans to find them on your next nature exploration.

Preschooler language development

Children of this age are developing more advanced language and communication skills: they can understand multistep requests, share stories in full sentences with lots of details, and may ask lots of questions. As you plan nature time, ask your child what they want to do and what they think they will see. Read books about nature and answer their questions (3-year-olds are especially good with why questions!). Be sure to talk about your nature time later in the day or as part of your nightly routine, and encourage your little one to tell others about their nature time. Have children this age sing their favorite songs outside, so they can practice their "outside voice." Let the outdoors be your classroom as you talk about colors, shapes, temperatures, and more based on what you

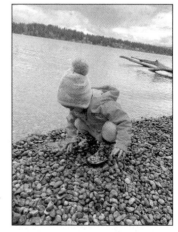

Enjoying a day of rock collecting.

ACTION ITEM: While most toddlers are open to eating all kinds of fruits and vegetables, sometimes preschoolers become very picky. Think of a way you can incorporate an outdoor activity with a healthy plant-based snack 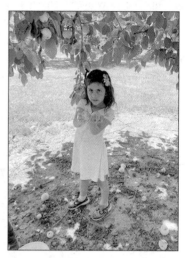 for your child of any age. Depending on the season and weather, could you visit a garden or local farm store with fresh produce? Could you not only plant some seeds for a fruit or vegetable but also eat one that you bought from the grocery store so your child can see the connection? How about planning a picnic or barbeque and bringing a fruit salad? If outdoor activities are not possible right now, you could share a story about a favorite food or recipe with your child and have them help as you grocery shop and cook together. Multiple studies show that children who help in a home garden, at school, or at a community garden, or even those who pick vegetables at a U-Pick farm, are more willing to try vegetables and even eat more servings of vegetables per week than children exposed only to the growing. We have had several parents report less picky eating in their children after they shared how vegetables grow with their children.

see. Try to come up with as many words as you can to describe something you see in nature (eg, the flower is *red, smooth, small,* or *wet*) or talk about all the ways rain is good for us and the environment. All this verbal interaction in and about nature helps preschoolers with their language development.

Preschooler fine motor or small muscle development

Picking up small bits of nature, sometimes called *loose parts,* helps promote fine motor or small muscle skills. Loose parts include small stones, sand, leaves, flowers, seeds, twigs, pieces of ice, stalks of tall grasses, and more. Although greenspace can be a big mown lawn, you will want to choose a less groomed place for playing with loose parts. The Illinois Early Learning Project has many suggestions about loose parts play. They encourage families to use loose parts in nature to spark their child's imagination while honing

ACTION ITEM: There are so many nature-themed books that are appropriate and fun for preschool-aged children. There are stories of animals or plants or just ones that include messages of exploring the great outdoors. This is a great age to start regularly visiting your local library and have your preschooler help pick out books they'd like to bring home. You could make a fun connection to nature books by suggesting a theme you both try to look for when finding books each time you go. *"Let's look for a book about farm animals today." "I wonder if there are any books about bugs!"* As you explore these books, make connections to your child's world, and ask them questions. *"Do you remember when we saw a full moon that looked like this?" "How many apples do you think are on this tree? Let's count them!"*

fine motor skills. This is because these materials don't have a predetermined function, and there are endless options for how children use them.

Preschooler gross motor or big muscle development

Outdoor time encourages movement, and as you may already know, preschoolers love to run wild. As part of your nature play, practice gross motor or big muscle skills. Encourage your child to run, climb with supervision, dig through snow, jump from small heights, and hop on one foot. Explore the natural setting you are in and all the spaces. Bring balls, kites, buckets and shovels, sleds, or tricycles to outdoor spaces to encourage the development of motor skills. Swimming in swim-approved lakes and rivers or walking in a creek should be one-on-one supervised at this age but is another great way for your child to explore the natural world and practice using their big muscles. Outdoor spaces provide the uneven surfaces that are so important for children at this age in practicing balance and coordination. Many children spend most of their time in indoor or curated built environments where surfaces are level, smooth, and pre-

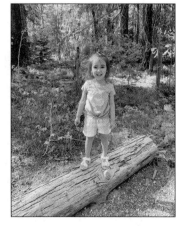

dictable, so their motor development is enhanced when they have to navigate physical challenges. Another emerging big muscle skill is the ability to walk along a narrow line or on a log. Try this with your preschool-aged child and

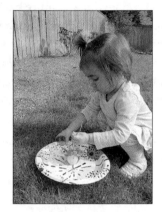

ACTION ITEM: Petals, stems, and leaves, oh my! Pick a flower, then have your preschooler take it apart—petals, pistils, stamen, stem, and leaves. If you have access to pansies, my (DG) 5-year-old granddaughter likes to pull off the petals and play with the inner part (pistil) that looks like a tiny girl with a long skirt or a king sitting on a throne. Have your child find small leaves, stems, rocks, or bark to create a habitat in a bug jar, then find a bug to move into their new home. Have your child give the bug a fun name!

Other ways to encourage fine motor skills with loose parts include

- ~ Picking out pieces of nature to bring home for an art project.
- ~ Planting seeds after collecting dirt in a cup; have your child use a finger in the dirt to make a place for the seed, then cover it up, patting down the dirt.
- ~ Having your child collect all kinds of loose parts and challenging them to make a fairy house or village.
- ~ Suggesting your child use all kinds of loose parts as food for their pretend restaurant or playhouse.

be ready to have them practice over and over until they can do it without falling off the log or stepping outside the line.

Preschooler cognitive development

Preschool age is the time of greatest imaginary play. Imaginary play stretches your child's cognitive development. You see the most imaginary play during child-directed play, but you can play along by being part of the "crew" for an oceanography exploration or dinosaur hunt or being the mama, papa, or grown-up bear creating a den for winter with your baby bear. This is the age when children learn to name colors, so use that in your nature play too. Math skills are introduced to children at this age so they can learn to count items. Sorting is also a skill to be encouraged and grown at this age. Nature is the perfect setting to keep your child interested in these cognitive building games.

Nature Nugget: Physical Literacy and Fundamental Movement Skills

Physical literacy is when kids have developed the skills, confidence, and love of movement to be physically active for life. *Fundamental movement skills* (FMS) are the basic movements traditionally associated with physical activity, and the preschool years are critical for the development of these basic skills. The most common FMS include running, jumping, throwing, catching, skipping, and hopping.

You can help your child develop these skills indoors or outdoors when they are given a variety of opportunities to learn and practice. Time outdoors is perfect, however, as they'll have the space and setting to do these activities and develop more complex skills as they learn. Your child can do these things in any outdoor setting, such as urban or rural, schoolyard or library grounds, park, or backyard.

When children develop strong FMS, they are more likely to feel confident and enjoy sports and outdoor recreation as they get older.

Preschooler social-emotional development

Social-emotional development in preschoolers includes noticing other children more and even joining together with other children in nature exploration. Encourage empathy in these interactions as this trait develops. You might encourage your child to take turns with others when looking at a tiny ladybug or help a friend find leaves for their collection. Emotion regulation is developing at this age, and your part is very important as you empathize with their strong emotions (frustration, disappointment, and anger, to name a few). This is called "joining" with them, as you acknowledge these feelings. Then you help them develop emotion regulation by "co-regulating" or "scaffolding" (suggest solutions or try slowing down; maybe show them how to approach the problem initially and then let them take over). The Child Mind Institute has many resources for parents about emotion regulation (https://childmind.org).

Nature play offers many opportunities to practice these skills, including when it is time to stop, or go in or go home, and your preschooler does not want to stop playing. For children who have a hard time with transitions, talking in

ACTION ITEM: Practice color identification with a scavenger hunt to find something in each of various colors. Or, if not so organized, just ask your preschooler to tell you the colors they see. Remember to look up to see "blue sky" and "white or gray clouds." You can ask about differences in size or temperature: "Which leaf is bigger?" "Feel how this rock in the sun is hotter than the one in the shade?" Take turns counting and sorting: "How many pine cones do we have? How many rocks? How many sticks? How many leaves? Let's sort them into piles."

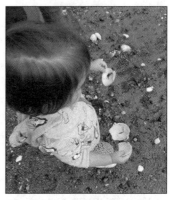

How many seashells are there?

Nature as a Tantrum Tool

A parent in my practice wanted to talk about the return of tantrums in their 4-year-old. Their child briefly had mild tantrums as a toddler, but as their language development improved, the tantrums resolved. The parent was caught off guard by these new tantrums and how intense and long-lasting they were. Often the trigger was something small, such as a change in family plans, a sandwich falling apart as the child ate, or wilted flowers she had collected the day before. The child loved her afternoon walks and they always had to keep going until they found flowers to pick. We discussed various strategies to navigate these tantrums by incorporating their child's love of nature and by checking out library books about flowers to read each day. We then discussed what happened after picking flowers and how that made their child feel. Within a couple of outings and wilted flowers, the new outbursts stopped and many of the others faded too. Four-year-olds with tantrums often express frustration with lack of control. This family helped their 4-year-old find something they could plan for and better control. Nature outings often give a fun and novel way to do this.

—Danette

advance about how long you can play in nature, and what it will be like when it is time to stop, can help ease this difficulty. If it is difficult for your young child to even get ready to go out, especially when the weather requires coats, hats, and gloves, make the steps of getting ready a routine. Follow the steps each time, calling them out or even making up a song about it: *First we put on boots, then we put on coat, then we pull on hat, and last we put on gloves!* Some families will even

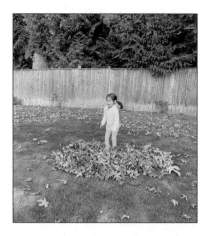

draw or print out a checklist with the routine and go through it each time with their child until it becomes habit.

Metamorphosis of a Baby Into a Child

The dynamic changes that happen from the newborn period to 5 years old are startling and such a joy to witness. Be sure to encourage your young child's development by using time in nature. Know that you are laying a foundation and putting them on a developmental trajectory for better health and well-being for life.

Nature and the Later Years: School Age and Beyond

Nature and the Later Years: School Age and Beyond

Your growing school-aged child continues to develop new physical, emotional, communication, and cognitive skills, just as they did when they were younger. Promoting your older child's continued development is just as important as when they were younger. Usually, schools and pediatricians will be tracking school-age progress, but you and all your child's caregivers can use nature time to nurture these developmental skills. You can find more resources with charts and parent questionnaires to track your child's progress on the Centers for Disease Control and Prevention website (www.cdc.gov/ncbddd/childdevelopment/positiveparenting/index.html).

School-Aged Children

Children of school age can truly explore nature with their new physical skills, improving judgment and relentless curiosity. At this age, they understand persistence and can enjoy nature in new and elaborate ways. They can start to be self-directed, experiencing nature on their own, and can help plan nature time tailored to their preferences. Your child likely has favorite activities they enjoy as well as opinions about ones they don't prefer. Collaborate with your child about your nature experiences, from simply experiencing and noticing the outdoors to going on much more directed educational or adventurous outings. Your child will benefit from both adult-directed- and child-directed nature play, so be sure to find time and arrange for both. At this age, you can still influence your child's preferences and encourage them to be open-minded to new activities or to try things again that they may have previously disliked. For some children, trying activities with friends that are provided at a camp or after-school program or planned by extended family and friends might get them to come along. Especially as your child approaches the tween years and naturally wants to spend more time with peers, finding and pre-serving an outdoor activity that you do one-on-one with your child or as a family may give you a special opportunity to spend time together. By laying that foundation now, when your child becomes a teenager and then a young adult, they might still cherish and look forward to doing that same activity together. This nature time could be as simple as an after-dinner walk or as elaborate as an annual backpacking trip you do together.

Children tend to be very busy at this age, enjoying so many activities that there is the danger of being overscheduled. Be on guard; non-curated nature time can be a good antidote if your child is overcommitted. As a family, remember that the time you spend together in nature will be among your child's most lasting memories, so keep it a priority.

School-aged children can make plans because they understand time and the future better. Their persistence and maturity make this a good age to try more substantial nature projects, such as making nature observations over time (track the phases of the moon or notice the seasonal changes), joining a community conservation project, or even taking the responsibility to grow plants or a garden. Children this age are more mature and able to wisely use tools as well. Besides gardens, consider making houses for birds or mason bees. You can find instructions on how to do this online or at your local library.

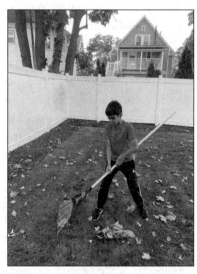

Helping the family by raking leaves.

Outdoor chores such as raking leaves, pulling weeds, or shoveling snow are a splendid way for your school-aged child to have more outdoor time while contributing to the family. Childhood experts report that children who

ACTION ITEM: Take a moment to think about what chores your school-aged child does now. What outdoor chores can you add to their current list? If there are no outdoor chores for your child, can they help with weeding or gardening for your neighbor or relative, at your place of worship, through a community group, or in some other public space nearby? For more tips on finding and setting up chores, check out HealthyChildren.org (www.healthychildren.org/English/family-life/family-dynamics/communication-discipline/Pages/Chores-and-Responsibility.aspx).

routinely have chores develop organizational skills and learn to balance work and play with improving time management. Successfully completing chores also gives children who struggle socially or in school an opportunity for success. Although it will likely take some time for your child to be good at doing their chores, be sure to be consistent by offering as much praise as needed. Other outdoor-appropriate chores include cutting the grass, tending a garden, washing the car, walking the dog, or sweeping the porch.

School-age communication and language development

Communication and language skills become much more complex during school age. Your child can tell you about their favorite nature experiences and why these are their favorites. They are reading and can choose nature-themed books. Even though children of this age can read independently, some families of young school-aged children choose to read together as part of a nightly wind-down time. On road trips, families can share nature books by having each nondriver take a chapter to read aloud or listening to a nature audiobook or podcast for their drive.

Another way to promote language development is to challenge your school-aged child to find natural places to explore in your neighborhood or during the next time you travel to a new area. Encourage your child to keep a journal where they can write nature stories, draw pictures about nature, or keep their nature observations over time. Keep track of birds or other wildlife spotted,

Family Book Club

One family told me that they started a "family book club" once their child became a confident reader and didn't want to sit and read with their parents anymore. They would take turns picking their next book, each family member reading it independently, and then discussing what they read. We love this idea as a way to nurture reading and relationships as your child gets older. You can choose books and stories with nature themes so those topics come up during discussion. A variation of this is choosing nature-themed audiobooks that you and your child can listen to together during long car drives if that type of travel occurs for your family.

—Pooja

look up flowers and plants to identify, or track tides or the moon. Younger children may need your help, but older children can take this on for themselves. For your older child, maybe their nature journaling can be part of a blog post or social media entry. This may inspire their friends to engage in more outside time as well.

Planning a nature outing with friends can also be a way to develop an older child's language and communication skills. They must solicit the wishes of their group and consider the skill level of the participants. Realistic goal setting requires that a plan be made around safety. Both goals and safety planning are adult competencies they must learn. The timing and logistics can be very complicated, so encourage your child to be realistic. They may not have all the skills yet and will need your help. Make sure you involve them as you solve each of the issues, to help them grow these skills.

School-age fine motor or small muscle development

Fine motor or small muscle skills are also blossoming at this age. Nature opportunities can be an inspiration for and setting to practice these skills. Drawing and writing can be frustrating at first, so your school-aged child may need your encouragement. Have your child draw what interests them in nature or use it as the backdrop for their imaginary world. Art projects using natural elements can become more complex with painting rocks, building small habitats for birds or bees, or even decorating their own fort. Snow sculpting begins with the gross motor or big muscle skills but then requires the use of tools or fingers to make the designs and features. Many school-aged children will attempt knitting or crochet or even needlepoint. Sitting at a window, sitting on your porch, or even taking these fiber arts to the park to work on a project makes them more fun. Nature journaling helps with language skills but happens through the use of fine motor skills. Also, encourage your child to create cards or write letters to a relative or friend about their nature adventures. The novelty of writing and sending snail mail can be combined with nature writing, or even pen pals. Older relatives enjoy this too and can help keep it going.

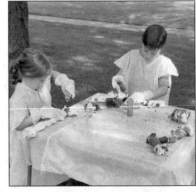

An art project can be even more fun when done outside.

Nature Nugget: Nature Cultivates Executive Function

Parents of older children are often frustrated with the last-minute or disorganized way in which they plan their activities. The areas of the brain responsible for decision-making, reasoning, and planning—processes that fall under the umbrella term of *executive function*—are still maturing throughout adolescence. For your child who is starting to make their own plans for outdoor activities, whether simpler ones like meeting in a nearby park or more complicated ones like a hike or skiing plan, use this as an opportunity to help them learn how to plan. Encourage them to think through timing and communicate this with their group. Is the proposed end time getting too close to a family meal or other responsibilities they have? What have they planned for transportation? Have they factored in time for traffic, and are they prepared for the expected weather conditions? How will they communicate with you if something unexpected comes up or they need help? Suggest that they make a list of everything they need to bring with them. Have them practice these skills on family outings too, so that, over time, they will become more skilled at planning and being prepared, which will make their outdoor activities more enjoyable.

Many children start to learn musical instruments at this age, which is a wonderful way to practice fine motor skills and coordination. If they are learning an instrument that is portable, suggest they practice or perform outdoors. Ask your child how practicing outside was different, including what they liked and what 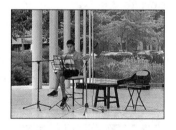 was difficult. During the COVID-19 pandemic, my (PT) son's guitar teacher held a recital in a community park. The weather held up and we were treated to some excellent singing and guitar and fiddle performances by children and teens. Although it was done outdoors for infection control reasons, many of us remarked that we enjoyed the setting and would love for outdoor performances to continue in future years.

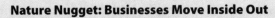

Nature Nugget: Businesses Move Inside Out

Kindermusik, a franchise providing music appreciation classes for children all over the world, flipped their in-person classes to outdoor spaces during the COVID-19 pandemic. This change was so popular with teachers and families that they have continued to offer it in many areas. Talk with your child's music teachers about doing more music and performances outside. Don't forget to look for community musical performances outside that your family can attend as a way to increase your outdoor family time. Pianist Hunter Noack offers family-friendly performances in parks and other open landscapes. The audience listens through headphones while they are encouraged to wander around and enjoy the natural setting. See more information at In a Landscape: Classical Music in the Wild (www.inalandscape.org).

School-age gross motor or large muscle development

School-aged children really start to excel in gross motor or large muscle skills. Running, jumping, climbing, skipping, and swimming are perfected during this stage and are often used in sports and competitive activities. Outdoors and nature time gives kids a chance to practice these skills and, often simultaneously, use multiple muscle groups. This is important because all muscles need to be used and grown in a coordinated way, not exercised individually, for the best development.

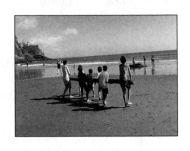

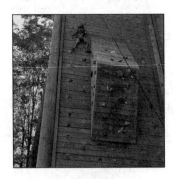

Older children experiencing growth spurts may lose some coordination and need to regain this. Muscle mass does not accumulate much, even with muscle-building activities, until height growth is nearly complete. Time in nature on hikes and climbs can be very helpful to build this coordination and strength, especially during growth spurts. Rock climbing, backpacking, snowshoeing, and swimming will also use multiple muscle groups.

Parkour is an increasingly popular activity where you move through obstacles (natural or created) by running, jumping, balancing, and climbing. Some physical education programs introduce this to children, or you may be able to find an after-school or summer program that enables children looking to challenge and test their motor skills. My (PT) children both loved parkour during elementary and middle school and their teacher held an incredible summer camp program where children practiced these skills in a large, nature-rich space.

Many children are still discovering and developing new interests at this age and may eventually lose interest in other activities they've done from early childhood. For example, some kids drop out of organized sports; if this happens, encourage them to find other ways to stay active. Even if children this age play a competitive sport, we encourage them to cross-train their muscles and engage in other activities to prevent overuse injuries. There is an increasing trend that some children focus on playing a single sport 10 or more months out of the year. We discourage sports specialization, especially before age 12 years, and instead recommend what's called "sports sampling" of different sports and other physical activities. Sports sampling is defined in the National Youth Sports Strategy (https://health.gov/our-work/nutrition-physical-activity/national-youth-sports-strategy/questions-answers) as the participation in multiple sport and recreation activities, with no single sport played exclusively for more than 10 months during the year. Research shows that sports sampling is associated with better fitness and motor coordination and can help prevent injuries. This is another good reason to encourage your child to try skiing, geocaching, disc golf, or running or water activities during a break from team sports.

Sometimes parents think a sport participation is enough to grow their child's motor skills, but sports often use just a limited set of muscles. Nature time is also interesting in ways that are different from a sport. Your child who may not be interested in sports may be thrilled to run through a park, pile up all the snow for a fort, and channel and dam puddles in the rain, while moving and developing their large muscles outdoors. Children who decide that competitive sports are not their thing at this age might still be willing to go on a hike or bike ride. With stronger swimming skills and water safety awareness, many children are drawn to water-based activities at this age. Also, think of backyard games or those you can bring to a picnic or barbeque: Frisbee, badminton, volleyball, Spikeball, cornhole, and more. These can also make great gifts for birthdays or holidays for school-aged children. These games can

Summertime Is Nature Time

Summer camps are a wonderful way to include enriching outdoor experiences and support motor development in your child's life. Local YMCAs, Boys & Girls Clubs, parks and recreation departments, schools, and independent organizations often offer summer child care, day camps, and overnight programs for school-aged children. Look for ones that include opportunities for lots of time outdoors and, perhaps, offer the chance for your child to try something new.

I knew I needed summer child care, so I would often try to coordinate with my children's friends' parents in the spring to sign them up for camps that provided such experiences. One experience that became an annual summer tradition for our family was Shoofly Farm in Sammamish, WA. My boys learned to care for bunnies and kittens, ride horses, churn butter, and make cinnamon-sugar toast on a firepit. We still have a pet black Holland Lop bunny, Mr Mysterious, that we adopted from this farm many years ago! After attending annually through the elementary and middle school years, my teens moved to becoming volunteer helpers and then paid staff during summer weeks.

If your child finds a summer program or camp that they really enjoy, you might encourage them to return for even a week or two every summer and perhaps they, too, would get an opportunity to build responsibility and leadership skills to later be in a counselor or staff role.

—Pooja

be a fun way to engage people of all ages outdoors, and you can dial the level of competition up or down depending on your crowd! My (PT) family has fond memories (and a few minor scars!) from an all-ages Summer Olympic Games—type event where teams competed in a series of outdoor games (everything from volleyball to limbo) for bragging rights.

Children with physical disabilities, either temporary, like an injury, or permanent, still need to move and be outside. See Chapter 4 for ideas about exposing these children to nature.

School-age cognitive development

It is very exciting to watch your school-aged child bloom with their cognitive skills. When they read and discuss nature topics, it becomes much more detailed and thoughtful. This aged child can understand and keep a calendar and help plan their schedules, including nature outings. Abstract concepts like space and time can be explored at this age and may become one of your child's interests. They may start to understand concerns about climate change and be interested in helping with reducing waste, recycling, and tree planting or other community habitat restoration. Does their school have an environmental club, sometimes called a Green Team? If so, encourage them to join! If they don't, have them look into how to start one. Engaging children in informal or formal community events where they can help with ecological or habitat restoration (eg, pulling weeds, planting, gardening) can help them develop a connection with the earth and understand their role in caring for it. Curiosity is important to develop cognitive skills, and many people think nature time is the best way to fuel curiosity. You can also explore groups or clubs that help children foster this curiosity and empower children through learning and civic engagement. For example, 4-H is a national organization that includes agriculture programs where children can gain practical skills in environmental science, agricultural science, and veterinary science, among other fields. We know children who connected with a local horse program and developed a deep passion for riding and caring for horses. Find out your child's nature interests and help them plan ways to explore these interests.

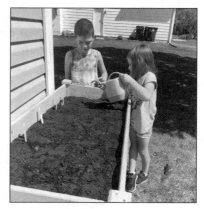

Nature games can be fun ways to stretch the cognitive skills of the whole family, such as using a compass or playing geocaching games. With their emerging computer skills, have your child map out a hike, urban or remote, near your home. Some school-aged children become so interested in computer or video games at this age that they prefer these games to going outside. As parents, we know it can be difficult but important to limit this preference. Consider using their computer interest with the outdoors, by blending both with age-appropriate games or apps that use the outdoors as the setting. These apps can help get your child who prefers technology back outside.

There are many virtual games that are played outside as you hunt for creatures; plus, some video game companies are now collaborating with local zoos and aquariums. There are also many free apps that help you identify plants, birdsong, or other nature, and even the online geocaching app is set outside as you hunt for small items left by other players. I (PT) recently heard about an activity called *orienteering,* which is a group of sports that involves using a map and compass to navigate from point to point in diverse and unfamiliar outdoor terrain while moving as fast as possible. Participants are given a topographic map, usually a specially prepared orienteering map, which they use to find control points. It's an activity that exercises the body and mind and may be the right challenge for your older child whether they pursue it recreationally or competitively.

School-age social-emotional development

As your school-aged child's cognitive skills develop, their social-emotional skills become much more complex. Important friendships develop and may experience ups and downs. Children at this age learn how to navigate friendships and can feel jealous, anxious, angry, or even sad at times. Being aware of the status of their friendships can provide you with teachable moments to help your child grow their social skills. Setting up playdates in nature or moving playdates outside can help friendships

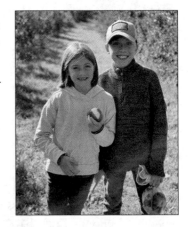

grow and can make things go more smoothly. Even then, you know your child's personality and might encourage activities that are not competitive to maintain a more positive environment and keep everyone engaged. Also, not all children have a chance to experience nature time, so being a nature mentor for your child's friends and their friend's family can have a profound impact on their lives (for more on this topic, see Nature Nugget: Nature Mentors and Allies in Chapter 3).

Children at this age still need their alone time, and young school-aged children may still enjoy pretend play. Parents in our practice often want to talk to us about how their children are making friends, especially if they seem to be having a hard time. Don't be alarmed if your child does not always want playdates to take place in nature; instead, encourage those who are struggling with friendships to consider joining outdoor activities. Clubs that encourage nature time are plentiful, such as Boy Scouts, Girls Scouts, or those organized by special interest such as skiing, hiking, or birding. Finding an affinity nature group in your community or nature groups organized for cultural, ethnic, or racial groups can inspire your whole family to find new friendships in nature. We know several doctors around the country who are leading their patients and patients' families in nature walks in a program called Walk with a Doc. Many of these groups have grown into their own community, expanding to include potlucks and other inclusive add-ons.

Nature Nugget: Parent-Led Nature Clubs

Parents throughout the country have created nature clubs. Some are informal get-togethers with a weekly or monthly walk, while some are more elaborate and supported by community groups, like parent-teacher associations or parks and recreation departments. The Children & Nature Network has information and support for anyone wishing to start their own nature club in their *Families Together in Nature Group Planning Guide* (https://eadn-wc04-796033.nxedge.io/wp-content/uploads/CNN_FTiN_groupresources_23-5-8_links.pdf).

The time you and your child spend together in nature has profound effects on their resilience in managing stress, on their self-confidence, and on their overall mental health. Nature settings give you ample opportunities to show affection for your child and recognize their accomplishments. We know how children open up, sometimes more easily discussing difficult topics while a parent is driving. This also happens in the quiet moments, while enjoying natural settings and outdoors together. Nature time gives you a serene backdrop to discuss more mature topics, like environmental responsibility, managing stress, and empathy for people living with hardship and our responsibility to help. Be explicit about your family values and why you have them, including right and wrong. These more mature, and sometimes difficult, topics are easier to approach in natural settings, so being outside also helps you have those important conversations.

As a family, volunteering with community groups focused on the environment or nature access can help your child grow in so many ways. Find volunteer opportunities that protect and promote nature as another way to model

Nature Nugget: Restoring Hope Through Ecological Restoration

With the mental health crisis facing young people, there is a specific kind of concern we are hearing about more and more: **climate anxiety.** Some national surveys have shown that more than a third of young people worry about the impacts of climate change.

While feelings of grief, fear, help-lessness, and guilt about climate change can affect people of any age, we are hearing about this anx-iety in children as young as those in elementary school. It will take some time for parents, educators, counselors, and other experts to learn how to best support children

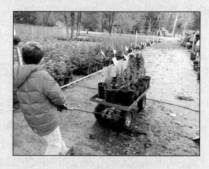

with these concerns, but we want you to be aware and prepared to discuss your child's concerns if this topic comes up in your family. One strategy that may help alleviate some of these feelings is to engage young people in ecological restoration work. Organizations around the world are bringing people together to elevate the connection between restoring our environment and improving human health. The premise here is that when young people plant seeds, remove invasive plants, or do other work to improve a degraded landscape, they are not only mitigating climate impact but also reinforcing their agency in being part of the solution. Even small actions can help restore hope, a powerful emotion that has been shown to promote action, health, and well-being.

empathy, building the adult competency of giving back to their community. In nature, your child can be a mentor to friends with less experience and fit-ness, working on empathy too. Your older child may be more willing to talk about complicated relationship issues in the context of a nature experience. You can talk about holding the line against dangerous choices promoted as peer pressure and making responsible decisions.

This is also the age to guide your child in learning from mistakes and how to bounce back after failure. While all these complicated social-emotional devel-opmental milestones are acquired, these older children are developing their

---

Playdate Intervention

My daughter has always been very social and treasured her playdates with many different friends. Around second to third grade, trouble broke out among the friends if more than one was over to play at a time. Someone was always feeling left out and feelings were getting hurt. As a parent, this situation is hard to navigate, so I found that sending the group outside to play really helped. A simple strategy of setting them up with a Frisbee or a nature art project outside or having them go to a nearby park to play on the playground eased tensions for the girls. I think being inside magnified the intensity of navigating social situations. Until this phase improved, I used nature time to ease the competitiveness for this group of girls growing their social skills.

—Danette

---

self-awareness, self-management, and emotion regulation. Nature tests these skills and provides an inspiring respite to reflect on past experiences and to calm emotions. Encourage them to turn to nature as a healthy way of coping with strong emotions and challenging circumstances. Keep talking with your child, keep listening to your child, and keep finding ways to support their social-emotional resilience.

Bringing More Nature to K–12 Schools

Children this age spend a majority of their waking hours at school, so it's not a surprise that this is an important place to increase your child's nature time. Many studies show that learning and exploring in natural settings improves learning, concentration, and behavior. We encourage you to assess what nature is in your child's K–12 school curriculum and if the playground has natural elements such as trees, bushes and flowers, natural landscapes, or a garden.

Whether your school-aged child attends a public or private school, nature in the curriculum and greener schoolyards improve the quality of their overall educational experience. The research supporting nature in schools is very compelling, and there are many resources for how to increase nature in this setting.

Nature Nugget: What Is the Best Age for Your Child to Have a Cell Phone?

Many children in the United States are receiving their first cell phones before they are 12 years old. This technology can be a mixed blessing for families as parents struggle with the pros and cons of their child having their own device. On the one hand, it can make it easier to communicate logistics with your child and be able to track their location when you're not with them. On the other hand, you may worry about excessive and/or inappropriate media use.

We highly recommend discussing these pros and cons with your child before they receive their first device and establishing family media rules right away (see the American Academy of Pediatrics guide to creating a Family Media Plan at www.healthychildren.org/English/fmp/Pages/MediaPlan.aspx). For these youngest cell phone users, it's best to identify screen-free times and zones such as no phone use during meals, during social events with friends, during homework, and starting an hour before bedtime. Many parents create phone-charging areas in a common space like the kitchen or in the parents' room so children are not tempted to check their phones when they should be sleeping.

If your child does have a phone, consider some of the ways you could use this technology in a limited way to encourage nature connection and time outdoors. You might feel more comfortable letting your older child go to the park or play in the neighborhood unsupervised if you knew you could see their location or have them check in with you regularly via their phone. You could have them use it to make sure they are back home in time or even use the timer function if they're taking an outdoor break from schoolwork or chores. You could also show them how to integrate it with nature by taking photos or using nature apps.

ACTION ITEM: If your child already has a cell phone, are there ways you can encourage positive use of the technology to promote outdoor time and nature connection? If your child does not have a phone, think ahead to family rules and values regarding technology use that you would want to instill. Set aside the time to look up the steps necessary to block inappropriate and/or excessive use.

There are 3 things to consider about your child's school.

1. Is there a robust nature curriculum for every grade?
2. Do they offer learning outside, moving instruction to the outdoors, and also hands-on outdoor learning opportunities?
3. How green is the schoolyard, and do children get ample recess opportunities to play and explore outdoors?

Nature curriculum

There are ways to incorporate information about nature and the natural world into the curriculum at every grade. This curriculum can include traditional science topics such as plants, insects, and animals; geology and weather; oceans, rivers, and lakes; moon, planets, and space; food chains,

Nature Nugget: Outdoors for All

IslandWood is an environmental education nonprofit in the Pacific Northwest that offers a variety of immersive programs to "help children, educators, and community members deepen their understanding of the world around them, explore important environmental issues, and see the power they have to make a positive impact on their communities and the planet." Programs include day and overnight environmental education programs for children, a graduate program and professional development opportunities for educators, and a range of culturally responsive and inclusive community programs to foster connection and appreciation of the natural world.

IslandWood is one of several organizations in Washington state that advocated for several successful state funding and public policy initiatives during the 2021 legislative session. These initiatives included over $10 million in funding for Washington Outdoor School for All, a project in support of residential outdoor learning for students throughout the state. This funding will help ensure that more Washington children than ever have access to education that deepens their knowledge of and care for the natural world.

Your state likely has programs like this or will be able to tap into federal funding expected to be enacted through the Outdoors for All Act by 2026 (www.congress.gov/bill/118th-congress/senate-bill/448/text?format=txt&r=31&s=1).

habitat, and adaptation; climate change; and more. These topics easily blend with other subjects to enhance learning. Examples include using nature prompts for writing assignments, counting and sorting natural items such as rocks and seeds, singing songs about nature and natural settings, creating art about nature or using natural elements, and learning about the history of space exploration. Many high schools also offer classes on environmental science, including Advanced Placement and International Baccalaureate courses.

Check with your child's teacher about how nature is incorporated into the curriculum. Additionally, your school, district, or state may support or even require environmental education in a more intensive way like overnight experiences. Check with your school district about their plans for teaching about nature and environmental education. More ambitious parents can volunteer to be on curriculum committees, or they can be chaperones for field trips, if this option is offered. After-school environmental or nature clubs can also be organized or supported by parents.

Learning outside

As a parent or caregiver, you know that when children sit for too long, they become squirmy and squirrely, oftentimes losing their focus. Just by going outside as a family, you can help them regain their attention. Some school teachers use this tool as well. If you know your child does well with this change in setting, ask at the beginning of the school year if your child's teacher plans to do this sometimes. Maybe consider offering to help facilitate this for your teachers, collecting small rugs, pillows, or carpet samples for children to carry and use to sit on the ground. For children who have individualized education plans to support their learning, ask whether something like this can be included to help them regain their focus.

Another advantage to learning outside is the opportunity to enhance the nature curriculum with hands-on projects. Some examples include facilitating a schoolyard garden or greenhouse that students help create, collecting natural elements for art projects, weather watching, and many others. Climate science and STEAM (science, technology, engineering, art, and math) topics are especially conducive to outdoor learning, and there may be organizations in your area that support professional development of teachers on how to integrate these subjects with outdoor experiences. Some of these larger projects may need parent and caregiver support, so also consider volunteering to help provide the physical help or fundraising that might be needed.

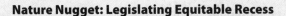

Nature Nugget: Legislating Equitable Recess

In Washington state, school recess was found to be provided inequitably. Surveys of parents revealed a wide range of recess time, from as little as 10 minutes to more than 45 minutes daily. Additionally, many schools withhold recess as a form of punishment or to have children complete academic work, neither of which is beneficial or healthy for children. State laws can help promote equitable and high-quality recess, but most states in the United States do not have recess laws. In 2023, a bill (SB 5257) in Washington state passed mandating a minimum of 30 minutes of daily recess for all elementary students with provisions for other recess best practices (including not withholding recess as punishment and encouraging movement breaks for middle/high schoolers). This was passed with bipartisan support in the Washington state legislature and signed into law. These efforts were led by the King County Play Equity Coalition that spearheaded the advocacy in collaboration with parents, educators, pediatricians, community organizations, and youth.

Source: King County Play Equity Coalition Action Team. Recess for Washington. Accessed May 13, 2024. https://www.recessforwa.org.

Check to ensure that your school provides adequate outdoor time before, during, and after the school day, with recess time being particularly important. Before-school opportunities can include support for walking or biking safely to school and before-school care that has opportunities for outdoor play. After school can be a time for your child to join a nature club or 4-H or be enrolled in after-school child care that prioritizes outdoor time. Children and teens learn better with adequate access to nature time and unstructured breaks. Physical education is important but cannot be a substitute for this. Check with your school district and make it a point to ensure that all kids are receiving adequate time outdoors, especially in nature.

Green schoolyards

Making sure kids and teens have enough time outside at school is not enough if the outside is mostly blacktop or concrete with plastic or metal play structures. How green is your child's schoolyard? Ideally, there would be many nature-filled spaces that feature nature-rich play areas, native gardens that attract birds, vegetable gardens and greenhouses, trails, outdoor classrooms, water play areas, shady trees, and others. There is increased attention to stormwater management in some parts of the country because of the increasing intensity of storms, so some schools are using this opportunity to turn stormwater capture into a nature-learning lesson for the students and even incorporate it as part of community efforts to manage stormwater.

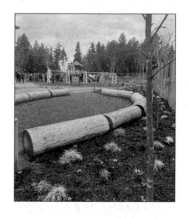

Another pressing concern is the increasing number of heat waves across the country; thus, typical asphalt schoolyards can become unsafe heat islands with temperatures more than 10° hotter on school grounds than in the surrounding neighborhood. In 2023, California's governor announced a new grant program to schools in the state to convert asphalt into greenspaces and plant trees to help cool the school environment. Renovated green schoolyards can support student's learning and health while improving a community's greenspace access and climate resilience.

If your local schools need "greening up," consider helping raise awareness about this issue. Community organizations; your city, county, or state; and local nature groups may all be interested in working together with the school district and parent-teacher-student association (PTSA). Some communities have been successful in fundraising from public and private sources for these renovations. The Children & Nature Network, Green Schoolyards of America, and the Trust for Public Land all provide resources and examples that can be helpful in advocating for greener schoolyards. You'll find information and toolkits that can be used to convince leaders and funders about the health, educational, and climate resilience benefits of transforming schoolyards into nature-rich spaces, especially with community input. Beyond the school day, these greener schoolyards can also serve as community parks if various community organizations such as the school district and parks department can enter into shared use agreements that allow the space to be accessible after hours (evenings and weekends) to community members. Depending on your bandwidth, bring this possibility to the attention of your school leaders or PTSA community or take on more of an advocacy or leadership role.

REFLECTION: Can you remember how you spent your recess time in school? What was the layout and what did you enjoy? Was there more concrete or natural landscape? How did the changing weather change how you played?

Sports and Nature

Children participating in sports are already active and, depending on the sport, may practice outside. But even children playing year-round outdoor sports need less structured, more direct nature time. It may feel challenging to find ways for your child to have both, so think about ways to combine these activities.

Consider steering your child to try sports that combine nature with sport. What nature does your child enjoy most: Snow and winter? Then consider downhill skiing or cross-country skiing, figure skating, hockey, or snowshoeing. What about water? Consider not just swimming but water polo, sailing, canoeing, rowing, or surfing. Wilderness? Hiking, rock climbing, orienteering, or cross-country racing.

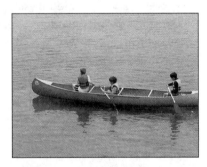

If your child participates in an outdoor sport such as softball or soccer, have your child get to practice a little early or stay a little late to incorporate independent play, by letting them run free on the field, or stop at a nearby park. This can also be a solution for siblings. Send them to an adjacent field for exploration and child-directed nature play, or to a nearby park, or consider planning outdoor free play opportunities with their sports

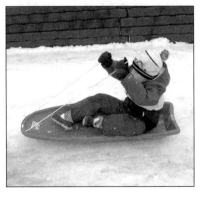

teammates. Share the job of supervising younger children doing nature play with other parents or caregivers who have an older child in the sport. Even older siblings can tag along and be employed as a parent's helper to supervise the nearby nature play.

Another way to combine sports and nature is by days of the week. If you are aiming for daily nature play, maybe on sports days, it could be very brief. Then plan longer and more elaborate nature time for the days there are no games or practice. This takes a little more thought and planning, but ask all

Team Nature

In our experience, children who play sports certainly love the sport itself, and friendships and camaraderie are primary reasons for them to keep playing. Children drop out of formal sports for various reasons, but an undeniable one is when they are no longer having fun. We have heard from parents and coaches that building connections between the players outside of practice and games is so important to maintaining a positive team culture. This may commonly take the form of meals together after competitions.

However, some wonderful examples that we've seen include parent volunteers organizing outdoor opportunities for the team to play together in an unstructured way. One of my son's soccer teammates hosted a team barbeque in their community park each summer for several years where the boys played pickleball and basketball and ran around together. We have also coordinated having the boys on the team go to a 3-night soccer camp in the summer, which involves not only soccer but also many opportunities for them to swim and engage in typical outdoor camp opportunities and foster their friendships. I've heard of other teams planning beach picnics, snow tubing, pool parties, and park gatherings to bring the teammates and families together.

If your child is in a sports team or another activity with the same group of children, consider suggesting or helping plan an outdoor activity for the children and families. Another benefit is that you get to know other families and may meet new friends and be able to count on them if you ever need help with your child when you can't be there at practice or competition.

—Pooja

the adults in your child's life to help. And, weather permitting, take other family activities outside, like eating and homework.

Finally, talk with your child's coach about ways you can help your child achieve a balance in their physical activity. Children are much more likely to experience overuse injuries in their sport if they do only one sport and it is year-round. It is better for your child's musculoskeletal health to be active in many different sports and physical pursuits. If your child is in only one sport, plan for active nature time so your child achieves this physical balance. Maybe the coach is looking for support from parents to help all the kids achieve balance or they may need to be convinced that this is important. You could also coordinate with other parents to plan fun outdoor activities for the team after a game or as a team-bonding activity.

Balancing time commitment for sports and all other important demands makes it harder to find time regularly for nature. Be realistic and realize that nature time may have to be more regular in the offseason, particularly for older children.

Looking Ahead to the Teen Years

As your child grows into the teen years, we want to point out that nature time will continue to be important for attaining the life skills necessary to be a successful adult.

While most of this book is geared toward younger children, nature time is vital for teens and their own goals for success, health, and happiness. Time in nature challenges teens to be their best selves, while providing restorative awe and wonder. Your teen will have definite opinions on what kind of nature adventures and experiences they enjoy and want. But these opinions change as they change, sometimes overnight. The great hike you planned for Saturday (and that you have enjoyed together for many months) may now be the last thing they want to do. Or they want to leave later or be back early in time to be with friends. Be ready to pivot and definitely try to plan nature time with input from your teen. Listen to what they want and consider what you know about them when offering choices for different experiences. These activities are really more about your time together and your relationship than the activity itself. Another

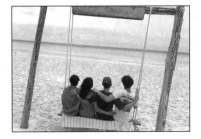

remarkable thing we have noticed is that outdoor activities that a teen might have shunned sometimes become a passion as they get older. I (PT) know several young people who were eager to go hiking or camping on breaks from college even though they may have rolled their eyes when their parents planned these activities a few years earlier.

Developing lifelong skills

We know you have many dreams for your child, and you want to raise them to be someone who is healthy, confident, curious, and surrounded by loving friends and family and someone who gives back to their family and community. And on that journey to success, you hope for them to make good decisions even when you are not physically with them to guide and nudge. Your child will also need to rely on the resilience you have helped them develop to face adversity and stress.

Sometimes it is easier to think of developmental milestones for teens as the acquisition of life skills. Their time observing and interacting with the natural world can help them develop many skills they need as adults. Some of these skills are competencies that need to be introduced and practiced. The way to guide a child to grow in maturity is to facilitate experiences and to ask questions, rather than to tell them or explain to them what they need to do or learn. Simple questions couched as prompts include "What do your friends want to do?" "Does your equipment need cleaning or updating?" or "How much time will you need to be ready for school/practice?"

The growth and development of your child into a competent adult does not proceed in a straight line but comes in fits and starts. Your role as parent or caregiver is to offer unconditional love and support, guide when you can, and offer opportunities for growth when you can, all while they are sometimes questioning and pushing back against the things you provide. Do not take any setbacks personally and do not give up. One of the life skills your older child may get to practice is having a job. There is an abundance of opportunities in nature, paid and volunteer, for older children to take on this responsibility. Former competitive swimmers may want a summer job as a lifeguard at their local lake or pool. Others may be excited to earn volunteer hours or money working as a camp counselor at a nature-based summer camp or after-school outdoor or sports programs. Our city parks and recreation department hosts for young children outdoor summer camps, and they hire tweens and teens to help run the programs.

Nature Nugget: Positive Peer Pressure

Encourage your child to be a nature mentor or ally for their friends or seek out that support for themselves (for more on this topic, see Nature Nugget: Nature Mentors and Allies in Chapter 3). We've all heard about the detriments of peer pressure on children as they may make their decisions with heavy influence of their peer group. What if we can channel "peer pressure" in a positive direction to encourage and support outdoor time? Ask your child about what sports or outdoor activities their friends enjoy. Could you persuade your child to ask their friend to take them along or introduce them to something they haven't tried or feel confident doing? Or, if your child has a particular passion and skill, encourage them to invite a friend or two along. I (DG) was successful in having my older school-aged children continue to attend nature-based day camps in the summer by finding a few of their friends to attend as well. Your child can gain appreciation for what it takes to teach someone a new skill, while gaining confidence in their own abilities, when they share their activities with a friend. We know kids who have helped their friends learn to rock climb, ice-skate, and use a paddleboard, for example. Even if it's not a more complicated activity, your child might be able to convince their friends to meet at the park or go for a bike ride, rather than choose an indoor sedentary activity.

Your teen's growing cognitive and executive functioning continues to mature into the early 20s. Planning nature outings with all the troubleshooting and logistics is a way for teens to stretch. Younger teens will likely need your direct help, but you can just check in on the plans your older teen is making for their nature adventure. Model (or learn together) how to use maps and a compass. Encourage them to check the weather forecast and plan what they need to bring accordingly. Have them help you put up a tent for camping or prepare bikes for a ride. Challenge your teen to research a nature topic to share with the rest of the family, then plan an outing together.

Goal setting is a part of cognitive development and is important for teens to practice. What are their goals for a school break, and how can they incorporate nature? What planning will it take? Will they need resources, and how will they budget for these resources? Household management, meal preparation, financial literacy, and time management are all adult competencies that should be part of growing competence in your child.

Older teens like to practice adult skills, so make sure your child learns water safety, basic first aid, and cardiorespiratory resuscitation. Nature time increases the need for these skills, and they are important life skills. They can be especially helpful if your child is baby-sitting or working with younger children as a camp counselor or in another capacity. See if your child's school or local hospital teaches these topics, or contact your local American Heart Association or Red Cross for classes. The American Red Cross has a class finder on its website (www.redcross.org/take-a-class/cpr/cpr-training).

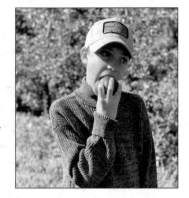

You might feel like the common ground with your teen is constantly shifting as they continue to develop new likes and dislikes. It can feel harder to connect with them now than when they were younger. Be on the lookout for clues about emerging interests and see if they may be open to trying some of these new

Appetite for Nature

As my son got into high school and especially after he could drive, it was harder to find activities that he enjoyed with the family. Parents in my practice often lamented their lack of success in getting their older teen to do family activities as well. Sometimes these parents even gave up trying. For our own family, I knew my son and his friends had voracious appetites at this age, and I noticed that if we had a large amount of food they enjoyed, we were more likely to get him and even his friends to spend time with us. He even finally noticed this and validated our persuasion: "Mom, you know you can get me to go almost anywhere with you all if there is good food also included." We found this was a way to increase his time spent with us, including during family outings in nature.

—Danette

A Different Kind of Birdie

When my son was 17, he discovered golf. No one else in the family really knew how to play or, honestly, even appreciated the sport much. He went out to a driving range with a few friends who had done it before and loved it. He then discovered a program that gave youth low-cost access to many local golf courses and was hooked!

Youth on Course gives children and teens aged 18 years and younger the option to pay just $5 (or less) per round of golf at nearly 2,000 participating courses and facilities throughout the United States and Canada.

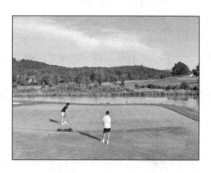

Their goal is to decrease barriers to access for golf, which is typically an expensive activity not easily accessible to many. With a set of older golf clubs borrowed from a family friend, my son developed this new interest and has loved trying the various courses in the area. Regardless of the weather, he said it's fun to be outdoors with friends playing golf and they've become pros at booking tee times and planning their golf adventures. He talked about the natural features of the various golf courses they've visited and the birds or animals they've come across.

While I didn't previously think of golf as necessarily an immersive nature activity, I have gained appreciation for this activity all because my teen shared his excitement for it with us. I now look forward to having the skills to be able to play a few rounds with him!

On a related note, did you know there are efforts around the country to transform golf courses that have shut down into public parks and nature preserves? What a wonderful initiative to repurpose acres of unused land into something of value for conservation and recreation.

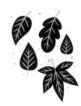

—Pooja

interests with you. It is important for the relationship with your teen to stay engaged. Some teens will be able to introduce you and other family members to nature activities they've experienced through school, summer camp, or their friend's family. One of the most satisfying experiences, as a parent, is when your child or teen teaches you something new. Continue to support their plans for nature time without you, because this is how they grow their independence.

As always, when they are setting out on a nature experience alone or with friends, make sure your teen knows how to tell you where they are headed, for how long, and with whom. Insist that they let you know if their plans change. Review age-appropriate guidance around making good choices, especially around alcohol and substance use, since older teens may not be supervised by adults during water-based or other nature activities. It is important to still be the parent or responsible adult even as their competence grows. Things can and will go wrong, mistakes will be made, and you need to be ready to help or support. They need this time alone to grow their competence, so encourage them in these outings. We both know that it is scary those first few times your teen goes out on an adventure without parental supervision, but nature adventures, with proper planning, can truly help them mature.

REFLECTION: Do you remember nature outings you enjoyed as a teen? Did you have nature adventures with your family? Are there some of these same adventures you can share with your own children?

Preparing for Future Generations

We truly believe the joy and awe of nature make the job of parenting a little easier and so much more fun. Just making the time for you and your child to be outside, enjoying whatever nature is available, is sure to help your child grow their developmental skills and gain the life skills necessary to be a successful adult. Know that you are planting seeds for the future when you see your children passing this connection with nature down to future generations.

Chapter 7

Exploring Nature-Based Activities

Exploring Nature-Based Activities

$\mathcal{T}$hrough these chapters, we have shown the connection between nature time and the health and well-being of children. We have mentioned activities you might consider while addressing the barriers to access for nature that we know exist. And, of course, what your child does in nature is less important than any time spent in nature. But we hope this chapter of in-depth suggestions helps create a plan for your child in nature.

These nature activities are only a fraction of the nature activities you can try. We chose these topics and activities because we found joy in doing them with our own children, and included are those that our patients and other pediatricians think are the most inspiring. Each activity listed includes information on how to adapt it for children of different ages or abilities. You can do an activity with all your children of various ages or adapt a beloved activity as your child grows up. We also included information about each activity so you can adjust it to fit the nature around you and your lifestyle.

We encourage you to check out nature ideas from other families, community groups (eg, parks and recreation departments, zoos, aquariums, Indigenous and Native organizations), and affinity groups (eg, bird-watching clubs; ecological restoration clubs; ethnic, racial, or cultural nature clubs) and through online searches. And remember, child-directed play is just as important as the activities you plan for them, so let your child's imagination grow outside!

Cultural Traditions

Family traditions are a wonderful way to engage children of any age, so we encourage you to lean into those of your ancestors, or create new ones for your family, that include nature. Many cultures celebrate nature with the change of seasons, and this can be an inspiration for nature activities. These cultural

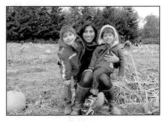

Pooja and her 2 sons on a pumpkin patch adventure!

traditions are sometimes available to participate in locally in many communities. Your family may have had their own traditions marking the arrival of the seasons, such as time planting together in the spring, outdoor adventures in the summer, harvest celebrations in autumn, and family gatherings during the winter holidays. For many years, I (PT) loved planting flowers with my boys on Mother's Day and looked forward to our annual pumpkin patch visit in October. Noting and celebrating the change of seasons, especially if you can do so outdoors and in connection with the unique features of nature that are specific to that season, will create lifelong memories for your family.

Rooted in Culture: Nature Inspiration From Indigenous Communities

Another place to gather inspiration for your nature activities is from the Native American and First Nation traditional practices or cultural ceremonies shared in your community. It is worth finding out about these opportunities in your area. If you don't know the name of a nearby community of Native American, First Nation, or Indigenous peoples, there are many websites that catalog these communities from all over the world, such as Native Land Digital (https://native-land.ca). Not only can you see the name of the Indigenous people, but there is often a link to that nation's website where you can learn more. Look up who they are, what they call themselves, and what the history is of how they have come to live in the area you share.

You may find community events open to the public to participate in ceremonies, learn crafts, and meet up to learn from each other. Some of the ancient Native practices are now part of ceremonies or even private, sacred rituals. For example, multiple tribes of the Salish Sea have come together annually since 1989 for the Intertribal Canoe Journey in the northwestern region. Each year, a different nation is the host, and all the other Coast Salish people join them for a potlatch tradition, a feast and gift-giving celebration practiced by the Indigenous peoples of the Pacific Northwest coast of North America. Preparations take all year as the families ready their canoes, practice their songs and dances, and make gifts to share with the other participants. The journey and celebration together take place over 1 month in the summer, and the entire community is invited to enjoy many parts of this celebration.

People of Japanese descent celebrate spring with Hanami, or Cherry Blossom Festival celebrations, with friends and families gathering under the beautiful blossoms to picnic and admire the trees. This rite of spring has spread across the world, and even in Seattle, people crowd around popular cherry trees when they are blooming. Another springtime celebration now found in the United States is the Hindu celebration of Holi. Traditionally, this is celebrated with having bonfires the night before and getting together with friends, family, and neighbors to shower each other with colorful powders and water. Many community groups, schools, and colleges host festival of colors celebrations, fun runs, and community dance parties to celebrate Holi. We hope you will create new nature-based family and community gatherings that you enjoy year after year. It is especially satisfying when you see your children enjoy the kinds of activities that maybe your parents or grandparents introduced to you.

> **REFLECTION:** Does your extended family or community gather for reunions? If so, how might you weave nature experiences into these traditions?

Exploring the 5 Senses in Nature

The magic of nature for your child's health and development comes from how a natural setting stimulates all your senses. What we call Five Senses Nature can be modified for almost any aged child with any ability. This activity can also be a way to bring nature to your child when on the go for busy families. You can look through a window when stuck inside or driving around, even rolling the window down to hear and smell when at a stoplight. This activity can also be done from an apartment, especially if you can open a window. On a recent walk with my (DG) grandchildren, we took turns calling out nature we could see, hear, smell, and touch while we

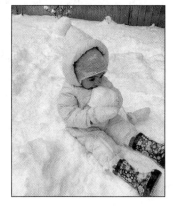

walked. My 4-year-old granddaughter became interested in the competition of finding another remarkable part of nature to sense. Doing any of these Five Senses Nature games in a rainy setting and in a snowy landscape makes the game fresh, with many different outcomes.

Holi: A Celebration of Spring

My family, in both India and the United States, nurtured in me a deep respect for nature. Growing up with Hindu traditions, I learned early on that mountains and rivers were often thought of as holy places worthy of pilgrimages. People made special, sometimes difficult, journeys to visit mountaintop temples or for a dip in the River Ganga. The sun, moon, and wind had their own gods (Surya, Chandra, and Vayu, respectively), and trees were considered sacred. Ceremonies and rituals typically included flowers, leaves, and fruits as offerings, and as children, we learned how to pick them respectfully.

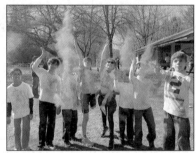

One of my fondest cultural memories from growing up in India was playing with Holi colors every spring, and I felt strongly about continuing this tradition for my children. Starting when my oldest was a preschooler, I would find a local community group that was organizing a Holi celebration in a nearby park and gather friends to join us. This became an annual event where we sometimes braved drizzly Seattle spring days to spend an afternoon chasing each other with powdered colors followed by enjoying a delicious Indian meal and dancing in the park. Even during the COVID-19 pandemic, I managed to organize a small group that met in our neighborhood park and played Holi with our masks on. I am delighted and proud that my children, who were born and raised in the United States, feel connected to this Indian tradition and celebration to welcome springtime.

—Pooja

Five Senses Nature for infants and toddlers

When you are outside, point out the nature all around. Show your young child trees, rocks, and clouds, naming these things in all languages you use at home. Encourage your child to say the name back or to point out some natural things to you. Naming or going back and forth increases your child's language skills and strengthens your relationship. You learn more about your child's interests in nature for other activities too. Then listen for a second and ask your child or baby what they hear. Describe what natural elements you hear, like birds or rain or how quiet it is in fresh snow. Take a deep breath and smell the air. Ask your baby to do this. Describe what you smell. Touch various textures such as hard and soft, rough and smooth, and warm and cold. Have your baby touch each surface too, and ask them to find more like it.

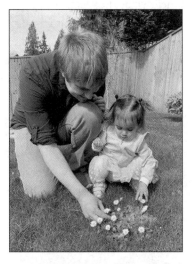

Taste as a sensation is harder for infants and toddlers to do safely. Are there edible plants or vegetables to taste when you are out? In colder weather, taste snow or raindrops coming down. Again, describe what you notice and invite your child to do the same. Continue to talk about what you saw, heard, smelled, touched, and maybe tasted later in the day. One of the most delightful times in nature that I (DG) enjoyed with each of my children and now enjoy with my grandchildren is when their bare feet touch grass for the first few times. Every time, each of them was at first alarmed, lifting each foot and trying to get away, but then gradually adjusted and even enjoyed the feel with their feet and hands.

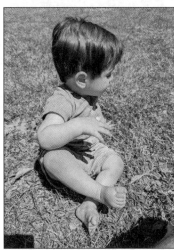

Not a fan of grass!

Five Senses Nature for preschoolers

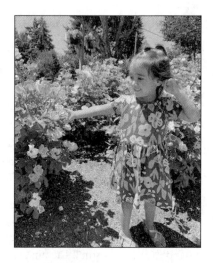

Like with younger children, you can take your preschooler outside and ask them what they see, what they hear, what they smell, what they feel, and, if possible, what they taste. Have them use a magnifying glass to study plants and bugs as well as rocks. Plan an outdoor scavenger hunt! An easy scavenger hunt in nature is to challenge your preschooler to find things by color: "Find something green, find something white, find something purple…" Bring a small bag or basket to collect and bring back home some of the textures to show other family members and talk about later. Your preschooler's collection could be several different rocks with different textures, or it could be many different weeds or flowers with different smells and colors. Encouraging them to describe these exciting finds promotes language and educates them on nature elements.

Five Senses Nature for school-aged children

Ask your school-aged child to call out one thing they see, one thing they hear, one thing they smell, one thing they feel that has an interesting texture, and, if possible, one thing they taste. Ask them why they chose these. Variations include asking them to write down their favorite nature element for each sense. Language, relationship building, and even fine motor skills are expanded. Be sure to have them use descriptive words. If it is safe for your school-aged child to go outside without you, this also works great as a child-directed activity. This can also be a fun way to compare nature in different areas. When you are visiting a new area, like a beach or the woods, or even traveling in a very different habitat, have your school-aged child record or write down their favorite senses from this new area. Ask them why these were their favorites, and compare this area to your area near your home.

A scavenger hunt for this age can be much more challenging: "Find 2 different mushrooms, find 1 smooth rock and 1 bumpy rock, listen for and identify 2 different bird calls, find 3 different tree bark textures, find ice and snow…"

There is a version of the Five Senses Nature activity for older children that is used to reduce stress and is considered a grounding exercise. If your older child is upset or anxious, or has had a difficult day, have them go outside and run through this Five Senses Nature activity as a calming exercise. This involves focusing on finding a specific number of things to see, touch, taste, hear, and smell. You will be giving them a valuable skill they may turn to in future years. Try practicing it yourself too!

Rooted in Culture: Onomatopoeia Fun

The Japanese language has more than 8 ways to describe snow, and many of these are onomatopoeias, descriptive words that phonetically imitate the sounds they describe. *Shinshin* is the word for the silence that settles into the world as snow falls. *Chirachira* is the word for lightly falling snow used in a manner such as "snowflakes chirachira." *Harahara* is the word to describe powdery snow falling down in a more hushed way. *Zakuzaku* is the word to describe walking on crunchy snow. Onomatopoeias are fun ways to describe nature, so your child may want to try to create new words for the nature they enjoy when using their 5 senses.

Walking or Hiking

Hiking or going for a walk is a wonderful way to be outside and get to some nature that is awe inspiring. Hiking is also easily adaptable to all ages and abilities, and it is often available to families in most neighborhoods, whether locally or farther away. A hike or walk can be adapted to snow by renting cross-country skis or snowshoes for a different type of adventure. National parks (and many other parks and snow recreation areas) have equipment for this that can be rented or lent out, even for small children. My children (PT) tried snowshoes once but decided they preferred to run, jump, and roll around in the snow in their regular snow boots!

Maybe your hike or walk can be to a beautiful spot, like a waterfall or a grove of trees. Check online to see if a local park is sponsoring a naturalist, a knowledgeable person sharing information about the natural world, to be at a beach or tide pool or another natural feature and then plan your hike to participate. Maybe your walk is simply a paved loop at a park or library.

Many communities have designated Heritage Trees to visit. These are notable or exceptionally beautiful trees that a community wants to honor or preserve. Try to find a Heritage Tree (https://americanheritagetrees.org) in your area or during your travels. Another kind of special tree to visit is a culturally modified tree. These are trees that Native cultures have harvested parts (like bark or specific branches) from, causing them to grow, now hundreds of years later, in a characteristic way. Find out if you have designated culturally modified trees on your hike by checking online or at the US National Park Service website (www.nps.gov). You and your child can also designate your own favorite, notable tree to visit. Hiking and walking are good for the development of gross motor or big muscle groups. It is good for your child's cognitive development when you plan your hikes and your activities along the way. Hiking also builds memories and shared experiences.

Infants and toddlers

Find a soft stretch of grass in your yard, park, or local schoolyard after school hours or a greenspace at your public library or place of worship. Place your infant or young child down onto the ground and have them wiggle, squirm, and crawl; we like to say they're going on a "belly hike." Laugh and roll around with them. If there is a small slope to this greenspace, that can make rolling even more fun. Even though this is not technically a hike, it is whimsical and outdoor fun.

Using a front pack, backpack, or stroller, include your infant or toddler on your walk or hike. For toddlers, talk about what you might see or touch while out on the walk, then point these things out. Be sure to narrate what you see, hear, and smell as you go. For waddlers or walkers, be sure to stop now and then to let them do some of the walking or even a little bit of climbing if there are low steps, timbers, or hills. All these activities promote gross motor skills and coordination.

Preschoolers

Visit any park near you, especially if the space has trails. Do an online search to help find parks as well as descriptions about trails or interesting features such as a creek or waterfall, a special view, or special trees. Keep the walk short at first to get a sense of how comfortable your child will be, but make the time walking longer each time you go, as your child builds stamina. They will be not only improving their gross motor skills but also working on their fitness. Provide snacks and water to help extend their participation. Making this hike or walk routine, by revisiting many times, can help you point out changes in the seasons or weather. Walking the same path in sun and snow are 2 very different experiences. Young children enjoy and learn through repetition, so be sure to add this to your daily routine.

Preschoolers are often interested in collecting. At first, they may not be very discerning (*every* pine cone they see needs to come home with you!) or even attached to what they collect (forgotten as soon as they are home), but it will keep them engaged while you are outside. One preschooler I (PT) know loves to paint rocks. When she goes on walks with her parents or nanny, they bring back a rock, paint it, and then return it to a new outdoor location on their next walk. Imagine the other preschoolers finding a joyful surprise when they see colorful and glittery rocks in their neighborhood!

School-aged children

Hiking with older children or encouraging them to hike on their own in safe greenspaces can also encourage a child's cognitive development through planning and organizing. Who will come along? How will your child make their way to the trail or park? What about water and snacks? Even if you will be going along, have your child participate in the planning. Backpacking usually means more extended hiking, including camping out overnight. This takes careful planning of routes, weather, food and water, and equipment. Look for gear libraries at your local library or community group if you need equipment and cannot purchase it. You can also check with secondhand sporting goods stores and online community pages such as Buy Nothing, Freecycle, OfferUp, or Nextdoor and Facebook Marketplace. When the local libraries have gear-lending packs for hiking or backpacking, many have found that it is school-aged children who check these out the most.

Another way to find support for more ambitious hikes is to look online for family nature groups and local park programs sponsoring community hikes. Other groups that may lead more complicated excursions include Boy Scouts and Girl Scouts, Boys & Girls Clubs, Sierra Club Inspiring Connections Outdoors, and community and religious youth groups. Be sure to check local affinity groups that lead hikes for children and families, such as Black Outside, Black Girls Trekkin', Outdoor Afro, and Portland POC Hikes. Check in your local area for groups close to you.

As some children become older, they may become reluctant to hike with their families. My (PT) friends and I would joke that the first question our tween

---

Surprising Stamina

No matter how much you plan, you can never really know how your young child will do on a snowshoe hike or during cross-country skiing. When my kids were 5 and 8 years old, we rented cross-country skis at a snow park. We chose a 2-mile loop to shuffle along; none of us had done much before and certainly were eager to try it. We thought our 5-year-old would tire out first and need to go back early. We were wrong! Our 5-year-old got the hang of it and sailed out ahead of all of us. Despite being dressed for the cold, my 8-year-old was not a fan of the weather, and eventually, we both turned in our skis. We waited where the trail looped back, and sure enough, my 5-year-old, with impressive technique, was still out in front of her father! Be ready for anything on your nature adventures.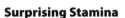

—Danette

---

children would ask when we suggested a hike was "Who else is coming?!" We realized that we would all have more fun and be able to hike for longer if we had their friends with us, so we began planning our outdoor excursions in this way. How wonderful that some of their childhood memories with their friends include outdoor experiences like hiking. I've also heard from patients and friends that sometimes hesitant middle schoolers come back to hiking as older teens and cherish those activities with their friends and even parents—definitely a full circle moment to appreciate!

Urban nature

A hike in an urban setting can be very different from a greenspace hike. Choose a natural feature in your city that is close enough to walk to, and map out an interesting route. In Chicago, the Bloomingdale Trail, also known as The 606, offers several miles of trail for bikers, runners, and those looking to ride or walk with friends or take their dog. See if your city has something similar. Sometimes buildings have rooftop parks that are open to the public. Often taller buildings and skyscrapers have a natural feature (such as an interesting sculptural rock, water feature, or tree) to note as you walk by. In downtown Seattle, many of the newer skyscrapers have public space open to explore. About halfway up the Russell Investments Center, through the back doors of a cafeteria, is a whole park plus greenspace accessible to the public. Interesting urban walks can already be mapped out for you to follow on city websites. Many Heritage Trees are in urban areas. If time allows, create a scavenger hunt made up of these interesting urban natural features for your older child and their friends.

Accessible hiking

Most national parks and many state and local parks note which trails are accessible to people who use a wheelchair, crutches, or walkers on their web pages. Take a moment to check these web pages before you visit. Some beach parks have beach wheelchairs for use or have installed beach mats that make it easier for navigating wheelchairs, walkers, or unsteady feet.

Nature Nugget: PlayGarden Inclusive Park

The city of Seattle has a beloved park called the Seattle PlayGarden: A Garden for Everyone, which consists of a park, a garden, a playground, and programs all dedicated to offering nature experiences to all children, including children with nearly any disability. Many of their fun, inclusive adaptations have been a model for parks all over the country. Check online to see if your area or state offers a similar garden or park that is safe and fun for children of all abilities.

Fun activities while on a hike

Sometimes your hike or walk is a means to enjoying other nature activities. The following suggestions are a very small list of the many things your family may enjoy:

Bird-watching: For very young children, point out the birds you see. Talk about the birds you hear and ask your toddler to find specific bird species. Pick up feathers and study their parts (make sure to wash your hands after handling these items!). Eventually, learn the names of birds you wish to find on your walks. Learn what birdsong you hear. Teach your child to use binoculars. If you don't have a pair, some libraries lend this kind of gear. Look into community birding groups that offer hikes and bird-watching, even for children. Have your child keep of a journal of what kinds of birds they found, where, and when. Read books together about bird-watching and talk about what you learned. Bird-watching from your window is also a way for children to enjoy nature from home if being outside is not possible. And it can be something you enjoy when going on car rides and out running errands.

Stargazing and sky gazing: Sky gazing starts as soon as you take your baby outside. Point out the sun, moon, clouds, wind, rain, snow, birds, and flying insects. Blow bubbles and talk about how the wind carries them away. As your child grows, have them describe what they see above them, such as the fluffy clouds or the airplane soaring through the sky. A nighttime hike or flashlight walk is the perfect time for stargazing. Count the stars and learn their names. Learn what planets you can see when using binoculars or at-home telescopes. Sometimes your local library will lend this equipment out. Try stargazing at the same time each week. Locate the moon and talk about the phases. Look for community stargazing clubs that invite the public to view the sky with more powerful telescopes. Visit a nearby observatory. Many universities have observatories with visiting hours for the public. Sky gazing and stargazing can happen while you are on the go, if you are outside, or if you are inside near a window.

Geocaching: Geocaching is the ultimate treasure hunt and is available all over the world. Using a GPS (global positioning system) receiver or mobile app on your phone and other navigational techniques, you and your family hide and seek "caches," or the simple items someone else has left, camouflaged, or hidden in an eco-friendly site above ground. Once you find the cache, be sure to sign the logbook, exchange one item, and put everything back like you found it. There are free apps that can guide you, and most cell phone GPSs work well. Libraries with gear lending may have the equipment needed. See Geocaching HQ (www.geocaching.com) for more information.

Citizen scientist: A good scientist is, first of all, a good observer. Encouraging your preschooler to describe the nature they see, hear, smell, and feel is a start. As your child learns to write, have them keep a journal to simply record their observations. This journal should contain whatever interests them, but on your walks or hikes, you could include observations about trees, signs of the season, number of wildlife spotted, or observations about weather or signs of extreme weather effects. If your older child is really interested in the idea of actually participating in research, the federal government and local universities sponsor and recruit citizen scientists. Some of the projects that recruit the general public include the Cascades Butterfly Project, your local zoo's community science program, the US National Park Service, or the Zooniverse platform that connects volunteer scientists with computer-based research to match every interest. These include examining images from deep space, studying whale songs, or monitoring remote seabird colonies. Also, check out Homegrown National Park (https://homegrownnationalpark.org) to join this international movement and share your nature observations in greenspace available to you. Nature apps such as eBird or iNaturalist allow users to contribute to biodiversity research. Many areas of the country host a springtime city nature challenge to record nature in your neighborhood.

Look up "citizen scientist" online for more information.

Foraging: Edible berries and flowers and even mushrooms could be growing wild near you and might interest your child. Find out what edible or collectible plants are in a public greenspace near you. Be sure to become fully educated about wild foraging by taking local classes or joining community groups.

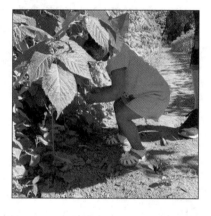

Habitat restoration: Many communities are working to restore damaged ecosystems. Community is often invited to participate in things such as beach cleanups, trash removal, tree planting, or invasive vegetation removal. Look for announcements about these opportunities in your community. Many Indigenous communities are important stewards of the land in their region, with much to share with their non-Native neighbors. A quick internet search will show you many examples of Native land stewardship and restoration and even large projects with several Native and local and state or provincial governments coming together to achieve environmental goals in your community. Native communities sometimes have wildlife departments, habitat restoration departments, or coalitions that bring many Native communities together for restoration work, such as the Lomakatsi Tribal Ecosystem Restoration Partnerships Program

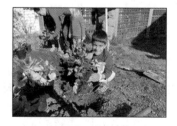

and the Inter-Tribal Ecosystem Restoration Partnership working throughout Oregon and northern California. Participating in local habitat restoration projects with Indigenous groups can teach your children about showing appreciation for another culture while appreciating nature. Look for projects your family can join.

May Day Baskets

When I was growing up, we created colorful construction paper baskets at the end of April in anticipation of May Day on May 1. We would collect flowers from our garden or neighborhood to put into the small baskets, leave those baskets on our neighbors' doorsteps, ring their doorbells, and run! It was fun to leave a basket and fun to get one too. Collect flowers on your hikes or walks near May Day, and leave them on your neighbor's doorstep.

—Danette

Safety

As with many outdoor adventures, taking necessary precautions to ensure safety is key. Always understand the difficulty of the hike you are about to take, especially with younger children. Make sure to run through various scenarios of how to react to unexpected situations and how to find help in an emergency. Know what the weather forecast will be, and always be ready for extreme weather. Check your child frequently for fatigue or other concerns such as blisters on their feet. Dress for the weather, and plan for unexpected extremes such as hard rain, snow, wind, and heat. Also, have a plan for contacting someone if you need help, and always let someone not on the hike know when you will be back. Plan for the worst and enjoy the best!

Nature Art

There are so many ways you can use nature in art or be inspired by nature for an art project. Art is also a great way to bring the outdoors indoors, all while still learning! Knowing the interests of your child helps you plan the best way to support this activity. Gross and fine motor skills are both encouraged for your youngest children, while cognitive skills are honed with older children when planning and implementing their art. This activity is for children of any ability and can be done in any season. Engaging in art projects outdoors "en plein air" was central to what impressionist artists did and something children can do in nature easily with watercolors. Take inspiration from the art of different cultures, including Native American cultures. Native art often features natural elements or is created in reverence of the natural world. Animals; the sky, sun, or moon; and landscapes are often featured in many artists' works, and some of these have even become iconic images in celebrating their cultures.

When time is short, always be on the lookout for natural bits to use in art later, even when going on errands. Keep paper and crayons/pencils in the car so your child can draw nature pictures when riding to or waiting at places.

Toddlers and preschoolers

Scribble tracing: Collect leaves, interesting seed pods, textured rocks, shed feathers, pine cones, and shells. Hold a blank piece of paper in place on top of the item and have your toddler scribble with crayons on the paper, over the item (so the textures are revealed). Have them use different colors with the scribble, telling you which color is their favorite. This activity will work gross motor skills as they collect the items and fine motor skills as they color over the items, and it will develop their cognitive skills with the color identification. Have your preschooler practice using scissors to cut out their favorite designs and glue those onto another paper in a collage.

School-aged children

Sidewalk chalk: This is an inexpensive and popular way to keep younger kids engaged while they get creative on a sidewalk or other hardtop area. Make sure they are safe from traffic or other dangers, as children this age may get

easily distracted. You can encourage your child to draw the nature they see around them or think about other colorful ideas, such as rainbows, cars, or abstract designs. In my (PT) neighborhood, I often see beautiful sidewalk chalk art with inspiring messages written across several blocks to welcome students back on the first day of school. Early in the pandemic, I noticed a small group of girls who would leave colorful art and cheerful

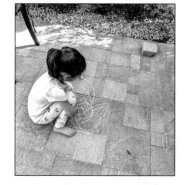

messages for their neighbors along the sidewalk. During the rainier months, I've also seen elaborate sidewalk chalk art under a covered gazebo structure in a nearby park.

Rock painting: Hunt for smooth rocks that are easy to carry or use shells you have collected that are 3 to 4 inches across. Using washable paints and small paintbrushes or color markers, have your child decorate the rocks or shells. Challenge them to use many colors and designs. You may need to help your little one plan to add more features after the first layer dries. Your child can display these new treasures at home or can share them back in your neighborhood. Decide which neighbors you will share these creations with, or maybe distribute them in your neighborhood or park. Challenge your child's memory by revisiting the creations during other times you walk near where they were left. Pine cones and larger seed pods can also be painted and decorated.

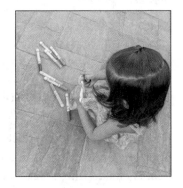

Sticky leaf collage: For this project, you will need to purchase clear contact paper and collect your favorite leaves or petals. Cut off a sheet of this clear, sticky plastic film; peel the backing off; and have your child place their leaves, petals, and whatever flat, natural elements they collected onto the sheet. Then cut another piece, roughly the same size; remove the backing; and place the sticky side down onto the art. Have your child create a frame that they cut out of construction paper or thin cardboard to highlight the art. Then staple or glue this onto the sheets. Alternatively, place the paper frame onto the sticky contact paper first, then add your nature bits to the middle, before applying the second piece of contact paper on top. As children measure and plan out the frame, they not only practice motor skills but also sharpen cognitive and math skills.

Flower press: For this project, you will need paper towels, a piece of paper that you want to mount the flowers on, lots of newspapers, 2 boards (you can use plywood or cutting boards), and many heavy items such as big books and rocks. Layer these items from bottom to top as follows:

- First heavy board
- First thick stack of newspapers
- Nice sheet of paper for the flowers to be mounted on

- (Carefully arrange) the flowers to be pressed
- A couple of sheets of paper towels
- Second thick stack of newspapers
- Second heavy board
- (Pile on) heavy rocks, bricks, or books

Wait at least 1 to 2 weeks before taking the press apart to check on the flowers. It is typically harder for younger kids to wait a long time, so if that is the case, you can consider gluing flowers and their leaves and petals directly to paper.

Snow art: Buy some food coloring and let your child paint away, creating pictures and designs, by squirting the liquid color onto the snow. You can make your supply last longer if you also have squirt bottles made from reused shampoo bottles or other household bottles; put the food coloring in, then fill the rest with water and shake the bottle up. The color will still be intense, but the supply will go further.

Nature photography: Digital cameras have made it much easier for children to take pictures. The instant gratification of immediately seeing a photo also works well for children. There are digital cameras specifically made for toddlers, with heavy-duty cases that withstand being dropped, but cell phone cameras work well too. Consider repurposing an old cell phone for your child to use for photography. Encourage your child to experiment with beautiful vistas or even whimsical, tricky perspective photographs in nature (eg, take a picture of a friend "holding up" the moon). Have your child use the photos to keep a record of birds spotted, wildflowers seen, phases of the moon, and interesting clouds and sunsets as a way to "collect" nature. Be sure to always ask why they chose to photograph that part of nature. Help them make digital or print albums of their favorites or use graphic design software to create digital art from the photographs.

Front or Backyard Nature

If you have a yard or access to close-by greenspace, this will be your child's first and most frequently visited outdoor play area. Many of the activities mentioned earlier in this chapter (see both Exploring the 5 Senses in Nature and Hiking) can happen in your front or backyard. Also, this may be the first greenspace you feel is safe enough for your child to explore nature on their own. This gives them the opportunity for free play or child-directed play and helps them use their imagination and creativity. It's also a space where you have more control of the environment and can pile leaves or grass to jump into or make mud pies.

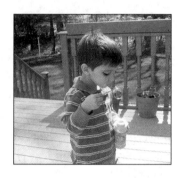

Here are some of our favorite activities and some ideas shared with us from friends and patients. See how many you and your family enjoy!

Gardening

Growing plants, flowers, fruits, and vegetables is available to every family. Even those who don't have access to greenspace to plant can consider buying flowerpots for a possible deck, balcony, or porch or even an indoor window-sill. For your infant/toddler, planting a seed or bean in a cup of dirt and then having them help water it can be their first experience. Keep the plant near a window and talk about why it is there. They will be delighted when the plant sprouts.

Growing Salad!

When my children were young, we had limited greenspace in our backyard, but I was inspired to have them grow something from seeds that they could eventually eat. I bought a large pot for our back patio and we planted seeds to grow mixed baby greens. My 4-year-old was excited to water the pot and he and his younger brother looked forward to checking the progress regularly that summer. Within just a few weeks, we had leaves big enough to harvest, and that was pretty exciting for all of us. More exciting than the planting and the harvesting was that my children happily ate salad for the first time ever!

—Pooja

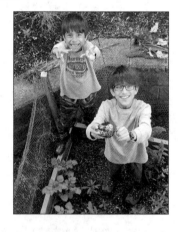

In your backyard, plant in pots or beds. You can plant vegetables or fruits or a flower garden, whatever suits your ability and interest. Ask friends, colleagues, or neighbors for suggestions on what grows easily in your area. Be sure to have your children participate in the planning *and* the work. Even toddlers can use a spoon or small trowel to work the soil. Your child can participate in harvesting and cooking of the grown food. Even if you do not have the space to grow vegetables or fruits, find a nearby farm with U-Pick options so your children can experience the joy of eating something freshly picked and cooking their own food.

Forts

Fort building is enjoyable for most children of any age (dare we say even adults too!). Sometimes these "construction projects" involve moving outdoor furniture around to make a space, while other times they're simply a tree house or an outline of a fort lined with collected branches. You can save cardboard boxes from deliveries and let your child get creative. With snow on the ground, snow can be rolled into big balls or piled up to create snow castle walls. If you have room outdoors, and your child has the desire, let them create their own personal outdoor fort to visit over and over. This uses their creativity, imagination, and motor skills. Ask them to show you around and explain all the features of their space.

Fairy or elf houses

Many children like to construct tiny houses or dwellings for imaginary creatures like fairies or elves. My (DG) daughter read a book in kindergarten about fairies and made several fairy houses. Give your child a space to create this structure and suggest some natural materials to use like rocks, twigs, seed pods, or acorn tops. You can even lend them some pieces from inside to use, like small boxes or containers, small bits of fabric or string and ribbon, or buttons. Be sure to have them show you their work once it is complete and explain all the parts.

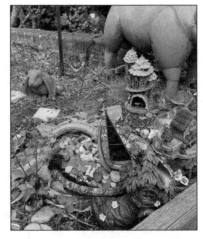

Nature Nugget: Nature Toys

Families have often asked us for recommendations about toys they can provide for their child. We know the outdoors provides many natural "toys" for your child to use in their creative play. But if there are going to be purchases or if family members ask for a list, consider toys that may compliment outdoor play: a magnifying glass, a bug house, fairy house supplies, kites, child-friendly binoculars, bubble wands and soap, an appropriately sized garden, digging tools, sidewalk chalk, weather-measuring equipment, flashlights, and outdoor game equipment such as balls and flying discs, to name a few.

Bug and animal habitats

Many young children are interested in bugs and small creatures. They like to find them in the dirt, on plants, or under rocks. Offer your child a clear plastic container such as an empty water bottle or clean sauce jar to create a bug habitat. Help them find what their desired bug will need, maybe dirt or a little water, sticks, or plants. Be sure to talk about air and make small holes in

Backyard Bunnies

I have vivid memories of finding 5 or 6 gray newborn baby bunnies that were nestled together and surrounded by grass cuttings in my backyard when I was growing up in New Jersey. My sisters and I would check on them daily and even caught a few glimpses of the mama rabbit. We dropped a few fruits and vegetables nearby, being careful not to disturb them. They were gone within a week, but decades later, I still remember how I felt: awe at finding these tiny creatures in my backyard, concern over their safety, and wishful thinking that they might somehow become our lovable pets. Your neighborhood may have rabbits, squirrels, deer, snakes, or other animals. This presents a great opportunity to talk with your child about topics such as animal habitats and how to safely coexist with animals around us.

—Pooja

the lid and explain why. Plan on when to let the creatures go to avoid having them escape or die. If your child is interested in the life cycles of insects, you can purchase butterfly or moth chrysalides to keep until they emerge.

Nature Games and Sports

Part of the joy in being outside is being able to play games where you can run and move with fewer restrictions. Outdoor or nature games can be a great way to keep your child engaged outdoors, especially as they grow older. Some of the best times for our kids were flashlight tag (obviously played at night), tug-of-war, hot lava tag, Frisbee, and other games of catch, hide-and-seek, snowball fights, sledding, water balloons, and more. There are many portable games, such as Spikeball, badminton, and volleyball, that you can easily transport to a park and play in smaller or larger groups. Some children really love competitive games, and others may have no desire, so you'll need to find the right balance for your child and make sure the activity remains fun for everyone involved.

There are definitely ways to make sports more collaborative rather than competitive for those children who are less likely to participate otherwise. I (PT) remember needing to create some new rules for basketball by restructuring our teams when our family's parents-versus-kids basketball game got too intense! Try other strategies such as seeing how many baskets you can score together, keeping the badminton rally going as long as possible, and keeping the Frisbee toss going back and forth. Of course, using sports and games as a way to teach your child good sportsmanship is also valuable, and they may find their inner athlete in a nontraditional outdoor activity or sport. Think also of cross-country running, swimming, kayaking, canoeing, sailing, skiing, and ice-skating. Look for community groups that help children participate in these sports and help them grow their skills. Orienteering is 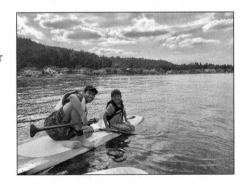 an elaborate cross-country race that requires participants to find the course. Most communities have orienteering groups that help coordinate these events or have a course open to the community. Look online for resources close to you.

For children struggling to get away from their screens such as video games or a computer, using nature or outdoor internet games can motivate them to be outside. Consider having them play internet games that look for specific animals or use apps that identify plants, insects, or birds. As mentioned earlier in this chapter (see Fun Activities While on a Hike), geocaching can sometimes be appealing to a reluctant child. These games use executive function skills and can often even involve their friends as well. This activity can also be a way to help your child attain some movement while having fun.

Community groups that support people with mobility challenges or disabilities may have equipment and resources to help these children experience these sports and games. The Miracle League, the Special Olympics, and other organizations offer adaptive leagues and opportunities. Check online or ask your child's health care team if they know of any near you.

Nature at Night

My son and a few of his friends participated in a brief game of flashlight tag during a YMCA youth gathering. These 11-year-olds had so much fun and were so inspired that they planned a big flashlight game of team tag in a small, wooded park near us. They spent days inviting friends and crafting the rules for the game. They had an absolute blast and played it several more nights. There are many other outdoor games played at night, such as shadow tag (trying to jump onto your friend's shadow created in bright moonlight) or flashlight freeze tag (when the opposing team's flashlight beam hits you, you must freeze until released by a teammate). Encourage your kids to create their own game too!

—Danette

Sport hunting and fishing

Many families go outdoors with their children for sport hunting or fishing. For these families, this is very important family culture. If your family never did these activities, but you want to try, look for community groups or outdoor sporting goods stores for classes that include children. Safety requires a thorough understanding of safe storage of guns (in a lockbox or safe, unloaded, with ammunition stored separately), knives, and other potentially dangerous equipment, and these items need to be secured out of reach of children, not just "hidden" from them. We have both had experiences during gun safety conversations at well-child visits of children revealing that they knew exactly where a gun was hidden. The Utah Chapter of the American Academy of Pediatrics created an informative website for families about gun safety (http://bulletproofkidsutah.org).

If your family is already experienced and safe hunters or fisher people, consider being a nature mentor for your interested friends. I (DG) remember fondly going out for salmon fishing with my grandpa and taking out a homemade rowboat with my dad on a nearby lake. Four generations of my family would go shrimping for the few days this season is open in the Puget Sound.

Nature Reading

Reading *to* your child and then reading *with* your child as they learn to read is very important for supporting their development and enhancing your relationship. Even with older kids, this can be a way to connect and carry on a tradition you started when they were younger. With older school-aged children and teens, you can also each read a book separately and then set a time to discuss what you read. For tips about reading with your children, see the official American Academy of Pediatrics website for parents, HealthyChildren.org.

Reading with your young child every day is a powerful way to promote language. Caregivers can be part of this too. Sometimes, for very young children, "reading" is quickly calling out a word or two as they hurriedly turn the pages: "Trees!" "Clouds!" "Mouse!" This age-group delights in reading (or having you read) the same book over and over again. *The Very Hungry Caterpillar* was a perennial favorite in my (PT) house. Ask questions and make connections with what is in the book to your own life. For older children, your nature reading can inspire talking about your child's interests in nature. It can even inspire fun activities for your family to plan in your next outing.

For all ages, reading about nature is a great way to extend nature experiences. For children reluctant to go outside, reading about an outdoor adventure may give them some comfort or reassurance, making it now easier to plan nature time. For families and caregivers with barriers to getting their kids out in nature, reading about the environment can keep this a priority. As children develop their own interests, reading can enhance their hobbies such as

Rooted in Culture: Nature Stories

The art of storytelling is an important part of Native American and First Nation cultures, and many of these traditional stories include explanations of our natural world. Children especially enjoy Indigenous creation stories, as they often feature animals and why they have certain features or actions. Sharing books by Native authors with your child is a way to increase your child's interest in the natural world. If you grew up hearing stories from your family, be sure to share them with your child.

bird-watching, art, and geocaching games. For your child interested in nature stewardship, reading may inspire more participation in habitat restoration. All children can learn from their favorite books, and we hope that some of your child's favorites feature a nature theme.

Our favorite children's librarian from the King County Library System in Washington created a list of books that include a nature focus and are diverse, accessible, and simply delightful. This list is a start but is not exhaustive by any means. The books listed here are written in English, but some of the more popular ones may have language translations available. Ask your local librarian about options for books in languages other than English. For the youngest children, you or another caregiver can talk with your child about what they see on the page and make up your own stories in other languages too. Of course, you can also share stories you remember hearing as a child or make up stories even if they are not written on a page. When I (PT) was growing up in India, my grandmother told me stories almost every night before bed. The stories were often about the supernatural powers of Hindu Gods or animal-based fables with moral lessons, and they have stayed with

REFLECTION: Take a moment to remember your favorite childhood books or stories you heard with a nature theme. What about those stories made them special to you? Try to find these books at the library (print or audiobook) and share them with your own children, or tell them these stories at bedtime.

me all these years later. Follow the interests and whims of your child as you and their other caregivers make nature books and nature stories available to them.

Book suggestions for young children

For infants to older preschoolers, look for books with compelling pictures, with short, interesting stories, rhymes, or ideas. For babies who like to taste and mouth books, and toddlers who are prone to ripping paper, board books work well until about age 2.

If you have access to a garden or are interested in planting a seed to grow on a windowsill, the following books might be complementary and of interest to your young child:

A Seed Grows by Antionette Portis is an award-winning book that goes over the stages of plant growth in a way that will engage infants to preschoolers.

What Will Grow by Jennifer Ward, a delightful and informative book about seeds and how they grow into different plants, includes always-fun foldouts for your child to lift.

Miguel's Community Garden by JaNay Brown-Wood is part of a series of books about gardens. In this book, Miguel is throwing a party and explores food growing, healthy eating, and garden flowers.

The following books are a great way to introduce using all our senses to connect with nature:

Look and Listen: Who's in the Garden, Meadow, Brook? by Dianne White will delight babies with rhythm and rhyme while inspiring your toddler and preschooler for when you can next get outside to play Five Senses Nature.

I Hear You, Ocean by Kallie George describes the sounds near an ocean, especially enjoyed by preschoolers and young school-aged children. Many children have never been to the ocean but will enjoy learning more in this sensory way.

I Hear You, Forest by Kallie George is a beautiful picture book delighting in the forest and focusing on hearing nature. This book can help you talk about visiting a forest or even a small group of trees with your young child.

Buzzing With Fear

My granddaughter had a beesting only once at age 2, but she became hysterical around any flying insects after that, shrieking "BEE!" She would often need reassurance that she could avoid bees when she went outside. For young children with fears in nature, talking about their fear, offering very frequent reassurance, and allowing time to pass are usually all that are needed to resolve this type of fear.

As adults, we can be mindful of the language we use to encourage curiosity and respect for the natural world. Why do bees sting? What is the role of spiders? Or worms? You could use this fear as a starting point for a conversation about the importance of biodiversity. We want to teach children how to stay safe while avoiding reinforcing unnecessary fears about the natural world.

—Danette

If your toddler or preschooler enjoys looking for bugs or pointing out animals outside, the following books might be of interest:

Thank You, Bees by Toni Luly is a board book that makes reading to infants easier, as they like to turn pages roughly and even taste books. This might also be a good choice for young children who are afraid of bees.

The Busy Little Squirrel by Nancy Tafuri, another board book, is about a squirrel preparing for winter. Point out squirrels or other creatures you see in your neighborhood or park as well as the signs of fall or other seasons when outdoors.

Nuts to You by Lois Ehlert is another fun and informative book about squirrels that is most enjoyed by preschoolers. Even dense urban areas often have squirrels, and many areas have different types of squirrels.

The following books offer exciting ideas for things to try when you are outside exploring. These characters or their adventures are very popular and compelling for young children. The adventures can spark your own plans for exploring outdoor spaces.

Baby's First Word

In my practice, I had a set of twins who spent much of their infancy playing on the floor by their sliding glass door and outside in their backyard. This yard had many, many squirrels that were unafraid to run up to the sliding glass door and generally kept the attention of one of the twins. Like most babies, one of the twins said "Dada" for her first word. But her brother's first word was quite delightful: "Squirrel"!

—Danette

Maisy Goes on a Nature Walk by Lucy Cousins is another in the Maisy series and a must-read if your little one enjoys the adventures of Maisy the Mouse. This series was a favorite in my household. My daughter always chose Maisy books when we went to the library.

Tiny, Perfect Things by M.H. Clark tells the story of a grandfather and granddaughter turning everyday outside walks into treasure hunts. This book might be good for a child who has a relative as a caregiver. Your young child would be able to relate to the sweet relationship between a grandfather and his granddaughter.

How to Say Hello to a Worm: A First Guide to Outside by Kari Percival is an award-winning guide to connecting with all kinds of nearby nature, told in a rhythmic way with great photos that is delightful for young children.

Wonder Walkers by Micha Archer is an award-winning book that points out the wonders of the wider world. This book would be especially good if your preschooler is having trouble coming up with something to do outside. It details the adventures of 2 kids using their imaginations to explore.

The Night Walk by Marie Dorleans is an award-winning picture book about a family adventure exploring nature at night. Especially if you live in an area where the sun sets very early in the winter, or only have time to do some nature exploration after work, this story can be inspiring.

Look What I Found in the Woods by Moira Butterfield, part of a series, is a fun and fact-filled picture book about the treasures to find in the woods. If you plan to explore a forest near you, read this book with your preschooler or young school-aged child to talk about what you might find in your nearby woods.

The Hike by Alison Farrell is perfect for budding scientists and follows the adventures of 3 young girls exploring nearby nature. This book can not only inspire children in their nature collections but also covers how each person has different interests. Good if you plan to take your child's friends on nature explorations with you too.

Outside In by Deborah Underwood is an award-winning book about nearby nature and connecting even when stuck inside. Enjoyable and inspiring if you don't have access to much greenspace or your child cannot go outside.

Finding Wild by Megan Wagner Lloyd is a beautiful book pointing out urban nature. Helpful for families living in the city to inspire exploring urban nature.

The Camping Trip by Jennifer K. Mann is a picture book about a young girl's first camping trip. This could be a nice introduction to camping or a way to reassure a reluctant child about to go on a new outdoor experience.

Wild Summer: Life in the Heat by Sean Taylor is a picture book and part of a series that highlights the seasons. Check out all the books in this series to start a discussion with your child about the different seasons and what you notice in your area.

Book suggestions for older school-aged children

Children this age will be looking for books that are compelling and readable, and great illustrations are a bonus. These children have specific interests but will be open to you suggesting new topics. The following list is a drop in the bucket. We urge you and your child to talk with a librarian at school or in your community to suggest more nature books that are to your child's reading level and interest. Books are listed for younger to older children, top to bottom.

Daniel Finds a Poem by Micha Archer is about a young boy finding poetry in nature. Beautiful illustrations. This book is inspiration for finding nature with your child in your neighborhood to inspire a poem or find poems about. Perhaps you could each write a poem about nature and share them with each other.

Berry Song by Michaela Goade is an award-winning picture book about exploring nature and the wisdom of elders. Every young child loves berries, so this story is very relatable. Definitely will inspire your child to look more closely at the plants in your nearby nature. Consider trying a new berry-based recipe with your child after reading this book—smoothies, berry cobbler, or some ice cream with berries on top.

The Secret Signs of Nature: How to Uncover Hidden Clues in the Sky, Water, Plants, Animals, and Weather by Craig Caudill is a picture book and chapter book for school-aged children to explore nature from nearby to far from home. This book is also a great way to challenge your child to look for the hidden clues you read about in their own neighborhood.

Listen to the Language of the Trees: A Story of How Forests Communicate Underground by Tera Kelley is a picture book, science book with a section to explore more, and parent/teacher guide with a section to help adults guide the learning of their children, all about the hidden world of the forest. Follow up by visiting a group of trees or a forest near your own neighborhood.

Citizen Scientist: Be A Part of Scientific Discovery from Your Own Backyard by Loree Griffin Burns is a how-to book for school-aged children to make scientific discoveries about nature in their own backyard or an urban park. Sometimes your family can be part of a local citizen-scientist group. These groups can be found online, or ask your local librarian to help you search for these opportunities.

Lifecycles: Everything from Start to Finish by Sam Falconer is a beautifully illustrated chapter book about life cycles and the processes of nature. After reading this, challenge your child to learn the life cycle of their favorite creature or animal.

Outdoor Science Lab for Kids: 52 Family-Friendly Experiments for the Yard, Garden, Playground, and Park by Liz Lee Heinecke is a manual for budding scientists to do fun and easy nature experiments in nearby nature. My kids were always drawn to kits you could buy to do at-home experiments. Use this book to satisfy your budding scientist with nature experiments.

The Backyard Birdwatcher's Bible by Christopher M. Perrins is a beautiful, full-color guide for beginners and experts. This is definitely a good place to start if your child is drawn to the birds in your area. Setting up a birdhouse or a hummingbird feeder could be the start of a lifelong hobby.

Mushroom Rain by Laura K. Zimmerman explores the incredible details about mushrooms common and bizarre, including some that have neon colors, some that smell like bubble gum, others that are poisonous, and more. Use this book to explore bizarre mushrooms in your own yard or neighborhood.

Nell Plants a Tree by Anne Wynter is a beautiful picture book about how a pecan tree that a young girl carefully tends becomes the center of her family. Maybe your child is less of a budding scientist and enjoys stories about families more. This book can initiate conversations about the trees in your neighborhood and speculation about who planted them, how long ago, and more.

Fatima's Great Outdoors by Ambreen Tariq is an illustrated book about an immigrant family on their first camping trip. This book helps illuminate new adventures in nature for your child, especially if they are fearful or not interested in being outside.

The Not-So Great Outdoors by Madeline Kloepper is a picture book about a reluctant camper who discovers that the (not-so) great outdoors can be just as exciting as screens and skyscrapers. Also relevant for kids living in the city who will identify with the lead character.

Eco Girl by Ken Wilson-Max follows a young girl as she becomes an environmental steward to celebrate her love of all things leafy and green. Many children are becoming passionate about environmental causes, so this book may be of great interest. Consider including steps you could take in your home to help the environment in your regular conversations.

We Have a Dream: Meet 30 Young Indigenous People and People of Color Protecting the Planet by Dr Mya-Rose Craig is a book that profiles 30 young environmental activists who are Indigenous peoples or people of color. Some children will be able to see themselves represented on these pages or at least be inspired by the brief biographies of young changemakers.

Diary of a Young Naturalist by Dara McAnulty is a memoir that chronicles the changes of a year in 16-year-old Dara's Northern Ireland nature. This includes mature themes, such as climate activism and living with autism. This might be a book for your older child interested in environmental causes.

Rebel Girls: Climate Warriors; 25 Tales of Women Who Protect the Earth by Abby Sher highlights the climate justice work of 25 girls and women from all over the world. The stories highlight their work as water protectors, philanthropists, authors, and conservationists. Great choice for your child who enjoys real-life stories and a wonderful opportunity to highlight women activists.

Nature Is an Artist by Jennifer Lavallee is a picture book that uses the whimsy of nature for kids who love crafts and drawing. This can be a starting point for your child's art or may help your child become more interested in the outdoors.

What's in Your Pocket? Collecting Nature's Treasure by Heather L. Montgomery is a picture book that celebrates famous scientists by exploring their own nature collections. This book is especially interesting to children drawn to history and stories about the lives of famous people. Encourage your child to start their own nature collection.

The Wild Robot by Peter Brown covers the adventures of how a robot survives in the wilderness. This would be a good choice for the child who is more interested in using technology than exploring nature or being outside. It can be a bridge for those children and spark their imagination.

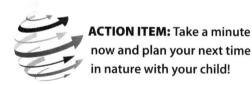

ACTION ITEM: Take a minute now and plan your next time in nature with your child!

Nature Is Never Boring

Boredom is uncomfortable, and as parents, we don't want to see our own children uncomfortable. We often work to make sure they are not bored. But handling boredom in a healthy way is an important life skill, only learned by doing. We have to allow our children enough free time to experience boredom and then encourage them to manage it. With all the digital media available, and overscheduled children signed up for every sport and curated experience, experts worry that some children may never get a chance to learn to manage boredom. This can be good for children, as it encourages creativity, fosters independence, boosts problem-solving skills, provides a break from overstimulation, and promotes reflection.

While we hope you use our book and suggested activities to help your child experience all the benefits of nature, don't forget to use outside, unstructured child-directed time as a tool for your child to learn to manage boredom in a healthy way.

Time in nature is the perfect remedy for boredom!

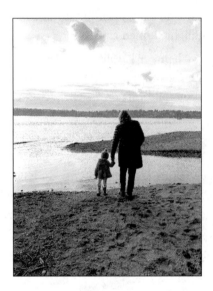

Planting Seeds for a Greener Future

Planting Seeds for a Greener Future

Our main purpose in writing this book was to inspire you to prioritize your child's time in nature. We've provided evidence-based recommendations and shared strategies other parents and caregivers use to engage children with nature. But we know parenting is hard work. You need to not only figure out what's best for your child but also ensure they have access to the opportunities and activities that promote their health and development, all while juggling multiple priorities and, sometimes, conflicting information.

Parenting Is Sacred Work

Even when we try our best to incorporate nature into our lives, various obstacles, such as a lack of safe local parks, inclement weather, the overwhelming presence of media use, or the societal pressure for children to be involved in so many activities, can all hinder our efforts as parents, caregivers, teachers, and communities. We've addressed many of these challenges in our book, including how to manage schedules and prioritize time in nature. There is tremendous pressure on parents for their kids to not just stand around—the pressure to get your kid doing something and/or everything! I (DG) remember having to make family rules about keeping it to one after-school activity per season…and that rule was as much for us (the parents) as it was for our kids, to keep from becoming overscheduled.

Our suggestions and ideas in this book are simply inspiration for finding nature spots and spending time with your child. Remember, we want children to mostly have child-directed free play in nature. The suggested activities are to help break down obstacles, coax a reluctant child, and find a way for each child, each family, to find their connection with nature. And remember to lean on friends, family, and others as your nature allies. We hope you use these ideas to create nature opportunities for your child and then shape those as your child grows and changes.

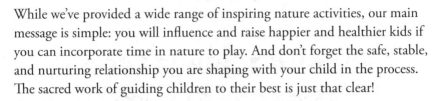

While we've provided a wide range of inspiring nature activities, our main message is simple: you will influence and raise happier and healthier kids if you can incorporate time in nature to play. And don't forget the safe, stable, and nurturing relationship you are shaping with your child in the process. The sacred work of guiding children to their best is just that clear!

The World Is Noticing the Importance of Nature for Children

Parents are not alone. The world is turning its attention to promoting nature for children. As we learn more about the importance of nature access for the health and development of children right from birth (even prenatally!), we are especially inspired by the attention this topic is receiving from international coalitions, governments, and organizations all over the world.

Access *to* nature and the benefits *from* nature on child health and well-being have been topics at the important United Nations (UN) Climate Change Conferences each year. The powerful UN Sustainable Development Goals have brought the governments around the world together to preserve and increase access to nature. Another important global organization dedicated to public well-being is the Global Partnership for Education. It has published a framework titled Climate-Smart Education Systems and has begun to support partners in shaping education systems around the world. The International Union for Conservation of Nature has put forth best practices for nature and environmental education plus supports the "greening up" of schoolyards. Look also for the UN Educational, Scientific and Cultural Organization reports on greening up schoolyards and implementing green educational curriculum. There are so many other organizations across the world taking on the issue of equitable access to greenspace.

One initiative that may already have come to your area is the national movement to create a local Children's Outdoor Bill of Rights in each city, state, or community. Cities, states, or communities come together to create an important declaration about outdoor experiences every child should have in that community. Some of these efforts have been established as resolutions, made into easily accessible programs, or issued as guiding proclamations. Examples of places with a Children's Outdoor Bill of Rights include San Francisco, CA; Austin, TX; Salt Lake City, UT; and Baltimore, MD. We are excited by the numerous efforts in progress at the local, national, and global levels to ensure that every child, everywhere, can experience the benefits and joys of being in nature.

Bright Spots

"Bright spots" refers to successful programs or strategies that have led to desirable outcomes and are highlighted to understand what makes them successful and how their success can be shared by others. Throughout this book, we have shared many examples of bright spots that are related to connecting children with nature and were built from family efforts, school efforts, community programs, and other initiatives.

We have heard from patients and their families about programs that have inspired or reinforced their connection to the outdoors. We have seen examples of educational, extracurricular, and community coalitions that have found innovative ways to connect children to the natural world, especially those who may face additional hurdles. We have been encouraged by local, state, national, and international initiatives, often resulting from cross-sector partnerships, to prioritize equitable access to nature.

There is so much all of us want to provide children as they grow and develop. The importance of early experiences and relationships that lay the foundation for lifelong health is what makes parenting and the care of children sacred. Nature can be one of the most powerful tools we have as we steer children toward nature exploration, connection, and experiences. As pediatricians, we appreciate you and are grateful when we can partner with you and your family. We want to empower you with knowledge, strategies, and, most importantly, hope.

In a time when it seems like we are bombarded with negativity, proponents of the bright spots concept argue that focusing only on challenges and barriers runs the risk of perpetuating them. These examples don't need to

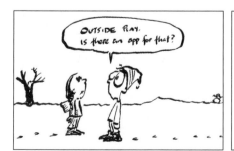 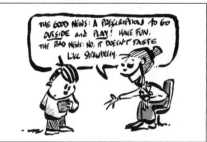

Source: Cartoons by Jack Maypole, MD. Used with permission.

reflect perfection but serve to shine a light on successes small and large and shift us toward a hopeful future.

We are filled with hope. Bringing all this information to you has made us hopeful for a green future with children, healthy and well from their time outside.

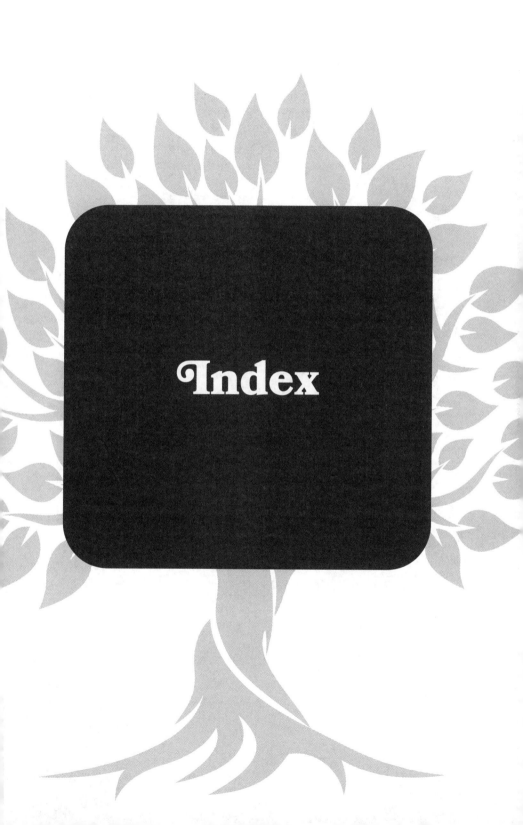

Index

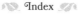